IN THE
DESERT OF ILLNESS

A Holistic Care Approach

Anthony Ade Akinlolu

IN THE DESERT OF ILLNESS
A HOLISTIC CARE APPROACH
Copyright © 2016 by Anthony Ade Akinlolu

Library of Congress Control Number:	2016938506
ISBN-13: Paperback:	978-1-68256-682-4
PDF:	978-1-68256-683-1
ePub:	978-1-68256-684-8
Kindle:	978-1-68256-685-5

All rights reserved. No part of this publication may be reproduced, distributed, or transmitted in any form or by any means, including photocopying, recording, or other electronic or mechanical methods, without the prior written permission of the publisher or author, except in the case of brief quotations embodied in critical reviews and certain other noncommercial uses permitted by copyright law.

Although every precaution has been taken to verify the accuracy of the information contained herein, the author and publisher assume no responsibility for any errors or omissions. No liability is assumed for damages that may result from the use of information contained within.

Printed in the United States of America

LitFire
PUBLISHING

LitFire LLC
1-800-511-9787
www.litfirepublishing.com
order@litfirepublishing.com

Contents

Dedication......................**v**
Preface....................**vii**
Acknowledgments......................**ix**

Chapter One
Understanding Spirituality &
Spiritual Care in Healthcare......................**1**

Chapter Two
The Desert of Illness **19**

Chapter Three
In the Hallways, In the Waiting Rooms:
The Pain of Waiting & Unknown Outcomes....................**33**

Chapter Four
The Desert Community
Home of Diversity & Community of All Faiths....................**41**

Chapter Five
Cultural Sensitivity & Holistic Healing....................**49**

Chapter Six
Holistic Care: Spiritual Care (The Chaplain)
& Medical Care (The Clinical Team)....................**63**

Chapter Seven
Care for the Care-Providers
Wellness of the "Desert Community"......................**91**

Chapter Eight
Spiritual Care for Cancer Patients......................**99**

Chapter Nine
The Twilight.................. **125**

Chapter Ten
Bereavement & Care for the Bereaved **169**

Endnotes.................. **189**
References & Consulted Works.................. **203**

Dedication

To all the patients, families, and caregivers I encountered in the course of my Pastoral & Spiritual Care career, who welcomed me to their sacred spaces amidst pains, discomforts, and vulnerabilities -

Thank you all for the trust!

Preface

The wholeness of a human person resides in the interconnectedness of the body, mind and spirit. They are dimensions that are integrally intertwined and inseparable without causing harm to the healthiness of the human person. Invariably, physical affliction can also adversely affect the mind and the spirit, and vice versa. In caring for the sick, it is imperative to care for the WHOLE person without separation or isolation of the inseparable dimensions. Focusing on an isolated dimension can be a disservice to the holistic goal of care that a care-seeker truly deserves. Without contradicting the gift of science and technology to human race, hospitalized patients and care-seekers in general often reach out for strength and support through their spirituality, practiced faith and religions. The mutual enrichment between medicine and spirituality has become an invaluable source of strength amidst the travails and the frailty of the human body. Healthcare Chaplains help to provide this melting-pot through their listening presence. They journey with patients, families and clinicians to help navigate the often delicate roads of hospitalization and the pressing challenges it often brings. These essential realities form the crux of this Book as I offer invaluable insights and great tips that can enhance holistic healing for care-seekers as well as integral wellness for care-providers.

It should be reiterated that as much as spiritual care for care-seekers has increasingly gained laudable awareness among healthcare providers, especially in nursing practice as well as integrating such valuable piece in physicians' training, addressing such vital aspect of the patient's need can be better addressed by trained chaplains. The competence and the expertise of chaplains, creditable to Clinical Pastoral Education

(CPE), would engender in-depth assessments that would meet both the pastoral and spiritual needs of the patient. This often recognizes the multidimensional aspects of a human person – bio-psychosocial (body, mind, and spirit) – while it enhances team work and professionalism in healthcare industry.

Savoring the years of experience in hospital ministry, working with patients; families and clinicians, I view spiritual care in the healthcare environment (or hospital communities as preferably called), as a need both for patients (care-seekers) and clinicians (care-providers) from diverse standpoints. While it would enhance holistic goal of care for the patient, it would, on the other hand, foster integral wellbeing of the care providers. The book, in all simplistic manner of approach, differentiated spiritual care from religiosity. This differentiation helps to expand the conceptual understanding of the subject-matter, broadens its practicality to becoming all-inclusive of a human person in its entirety. This researched piece brings to fore the humanness of physicians and clinicians in general. It encourages care providers to embrace their vulnerability and the magnitude of their human feelings. That is, the practice of authentic medicine and the care of one's spiritual wellness are not mutually exclusive. Rather, they stand as mutual enhancements, increasing the chances of patient safety and care. This experiential discovery hearts this work.

This revised edition considers a major contributory element to achieving holistic goal of care – cultural sensitivity. Effective outcome of health care delivery is underscored by the practice of awareness, sensitivity, and the demonstration of understanding, as well as the integration of cultural values of the patients. Insensitivity to cultural values or the failure to integrate such esteemed cultural values into the health care service delivery may inadvertently compromise good and quality outcome. Consequently, I consider the role of cultural sensitivity in holistic care approach to be pricey if omitted from this book.

In all ramifications, this text, a culmination of more than 10 years of caring for the sick, demonstrates the greater and timely results that can be achieved when spiritual care assessments and the involvement of a chaplain are initiated from the onset and not at sunset. In the arid desert of illness, patients often thirst for comforting hands; soothing voice of hope; listening and non-judgmental presence; help when feeling helpless; companion when feeling alone; Divine presence when feeling abandoned; and, spiritual guidance when at crossroads.

Anthony Ade Akinlolu, MBA, MA, BCC

Acknowledgments

This second edition could not have been possible if not for the generous support of kind hearted people. Above all, I am eternally indebted to all the patients that afforded me the invaluable privilege to learn from their unique stories and life experiences. With every sense of deepest appreciation, I acknowledge all the nursing units at MedStar Washington Hospital Center that hosted my facilitated in-service lectures/trainings which form the bedrock for this book. The same goes to acknowledging the wonderful nurses, resident-doctors, and leadership colleagues for seeing and promoting the value of holistic healing in our hospital community. Every forum created through your professional support sharpens the conceptual perspectives expressed in this book. You are all valued and exceptional team!

I also acknowledge great Minds that have taken on the challenge of expanding the frontier of knowledge and understanding on the essential needs for spiritual care in view of holistic healing in the arena of medicine, especially those whose brilliant works, published or in-press, are cited in this Book. Every achieved goal and realized dream must have passed through the gates of some or many encouragers – every help, every word of encouragement, and every constructive feedback are immensely appreciated!

Prayer for Desert Times

The Journeys of our lives are never fully charted.
There come, sometimes, to each of us, deserts to cross,
barren stretches
where the green edge on the horizon may be our destination,
or an oasis on our way,
or a mirage that beckons and will leave us lost.
When fear grips the heart, or despair bows the head,
may we bend as heart and head lead us down
to touch the ground beneath our feet,
and scoop some sand into our hands,
and receive what the sand would teach us:
It holds the warmth of the sun when the sun has left our sight,
as it holds the cool of the night when the stars have faded.
And hidden among its grains are tiny seeds, at rest and waiting.
Dormant, yet undefeated. Desert flowers.
They endure.
Moistened by our tears,
and by the rain that comes to end even the longest drought,
they send down roots, and they bloom.
Oh, may we believe in those seeds,
and the seeds within us.
May we remember in our dry seasons
that we, too, are desert flowers.
Amen.

-Margaret Keip

(Source: L. Annie Foerster, 'For Praying Out Loud: Interfaith Prayers for Public Occasions' 2003)

Chapter One

Understanding Spirituality & Spiritual Care in Healthcare

"The lesson which life repeats and constantly enforces is... Look underfoot You are always nearer the divine and the true sources of your power than you think."
— *John Burroughs 1887 - 1921*

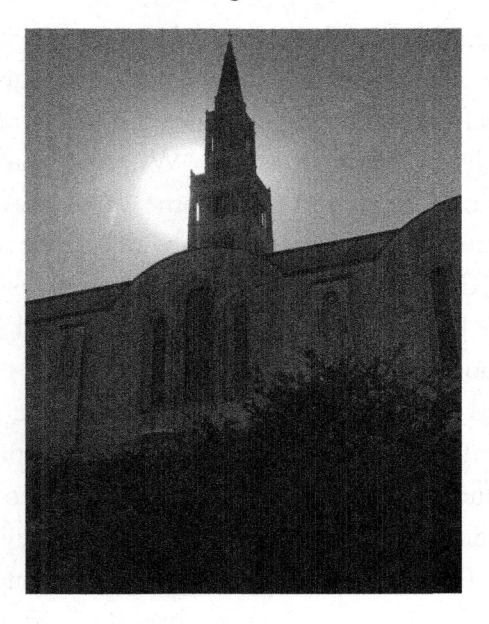

What has spirituality got to do with medicine? What a legitimate question! But you may soon find out. This is a foundation chapter. The entire book will be premised on a good and solid conceptual understanding of 'Spirituality' although without attempting to make it a book on 'spirituality.' With that being said, it is my intention, in this Chapter, to discuss the following: 'Spirituality' – what it is and what it's not, 'What is Pastoral Care?' 'How is Pastoral Care different from Spiritual Care?' 'What are the four "*Must-Know*" realities and expectations about hospitalization?' 'What are the expectations of a chaplain's or a clergy's holistic pastoral/spiritual care visit to the sick?' and 'How does the typical daily pastoral engagement of the chaplain look like in a clinical environment?'

As I stopped by to visit Mr. Z, in the course of my daily rounds, along with his 'good morning,' he quickly said to me, "Oh Father, I'm not religious but I'm a spiritual person." Some have been more explicit in similar responses: "Oh, I'm not a good Catholic…I don't go to church every Sunday…but I'm spiritual…" Some nurses or doctors would add, when placing a consult, 'I'm not sure if s/he is religious, but s/he appears spiritual.' This subtle "tension" not only exists in a descriptive manner, it also, somehow, shapes how a chaplain is perceived or understood as well as what a chaplain understands his/her roles to be.

One of the four hospitals I've been a part of featured Bioethics and Spiritual Care disciplines. During a surgical Grand Rounds, a chief ICU (Intensive Care Unit) Physician asked, "When is it appropriate to call you guys [chaplains]? I see you guys come in to pray when a patient is deceased…" The surgeon was probably not alone in that arena of "misconception." Chaplains have often been seen as "prayer people." This might rightly be so. However, this depicts limited understanding of the roles and responsibilities of chaplains to patients, families, staff and the entire hospital community. The calming presence of chaplains, for instance, speaks volumes without necessarily uttering prayers.

To further our enlightenment, it is imperative to address lines of distinction between "religiosity" and "spirituality." They might sound or appear similar, yet they are not exactly the same. Although both concepts could semantically be used interchangeably and might have been applied to depict the same understanding; yet, they are quite distinct in practical application. Hence, it is very crucial to discuss the differences between these two concepts that chaplains or healthcare workers often confront as they strive to provide the holistic goal of care to their patients. These differences, regardless of subtlety, consist in the nature of services provided for the recipients – patients. For the purpose of this book and in order to distinctly capture the roles of chaplains in the hospital, therefore, the concepts will be differentiated.

Spirituality – What It Is Not

Sifting through what 'spirituality' is and what it is not, it is necessary to begin by using the principle of elimination or negation separating the chaff from the wheat. Thus, 'spirituality' is:

- Not **ONLY** about belief systems or devout practices.
- Not **SIMPLY** about religiousness or religiosity – how religious is the individual/patient
- Not **NECESSARILY** about piety – how sanctimonious, virtuous or impious?
- Not **CONFINED** to organized religion or religious affiliation – Do you or how often do you go to synagogue, assembly, church, mosque, or belong to any worship group?
- Finally, Not **RESTRICTED** to "Where?" or a place of worship.

Spiritual care, as clearly illustrated above, will not be considered, as such, if it does not encompass more than the tenets of religious practices and confinements. Cramping such varsatile care to any of the above-highlighted categories will be to minimally understand what spiritual care fully comprises of.

What Is Spirituality & Spiritual Care?

Now that we know that 'spiritual care' is not simply or necessarily confined to structured sets of belief systems or pious practices, it is then appropriate to confront the central focus of this chapter: 'what then is spirituality?'

Spirituality involves the *totality* of the human person in relation to the Divine, the Supreme Being, the Transcendent – known – by different worthy names as God, Allah, Yahweh, Deity, Brahman, Krishna, Buddha, just to mention a few. It involves the existing personal relationship between a human person and the Transcendent. Reviewing what experts and great authors have written about "Spirituality" would be a wise start. Hands and Fehr (1993) opine that spirituality entails a concrete way an individual person lives cognizant of their relationship to the mystery of God. Corroborating the idea that spirituality connects the human person to the divine, Amenta opines that, "the spiritual is the self, or I, the essence of personhood, the God within, that part which communes with the transcendent. It is that part of each individual which longs for ultimate awareness, meaning, value, purpose, beauty, dignity, relatedness, and integrity."[1] Spirituality, a personal relationship with the Divine or Supreme Being, also includes how this relationship confronts or is challenged by existential "test" or "trial" in the real world.

As used in the "Cultural & Spiritual Sensitivity – A Learning Module for Health Care Professionals" developed by the Pastoral Care Leadership and Practice Group of Health Care Chaplaincy, a revision and an update of earlier work by Susan Wintz and Earl Cooper, spirituality would refer to "our inner belief system. It is a delicate 'spirit-to-spirit' relationship to oneself, others, and the God of one's understanding."[2] For Stoll, "Spirituality is my being; my inner person. It is who I am – unique and alive. It is me expressed through my body, my thinking, my feelings, my judgments, and my creativity. My spirituality motivates me to choose meaningful relationships and pursuits…I respond to and appreciate God, other people, a sunset, a symphony, and spring…Spirituality allows me to reflect on myself… and enable s me to value, to worship, and to communicate with the holy, the transcendent."[3]

"Spirituality is a personal search for meaning and purpose in life, which may or may not be related to religion. It entails connection to self-chosen and or religious beliefs, values and practices that give meaning to life, thereby inspiring and motivating individuals to achieve their optimal being. This connection brings faith, hope, peace and empowerment. The results are joy, forgiveness of oneself and others, awareness and acceptance of hardship and mortality, a heightened sense of physical and emotional well-being, and the ability to transcend beyond the infirmities of existence."[4] It is evident, from the above definitions that 'spirituality' would encompass the whole of the human person in entirety. Spiritual care, therefore, would mean 'caring for the whole of the human person.' Spiritual needs "involve finding meaning in one's life and ending disagreements with others, if possible."[5] In other words, spiritual care aims at restoring the intra-connection first, within 'the self.' Second, it seeks to foster interconnection with others. Both intra and interconnectedness are aimed at achieving wholeness, completeness, and inner peace that will contribute to the overall holistic care of the care seeker. Reed succinctly captured the crux of spirituality as both "intra" and "inter" when opined that spirituality is the "interconnectedness, within the individual, the environment, and with a transcendent being."[6]

When contextualized within the discourse of this book, that is, from the perspective of the invaluable importance of spiritual care in the overall holistic goal of care that a care seeker should receive, spirituality as a subject-matter is even more enriched in the words of David Kelly: "The human person is an embodied spirit, an animated body, and so human health involves spiritual and physical aspects in inseparable interaction."[7] In fact, Kelly further contends that the complete separation of the human person into spiritual and physical componential entities can be detrimental.

In contradistinction, religion "refers to the externals of our belief system: church, prayers, traditions, rites, rituals, etc."[8] Thus, 'religiousness' refers to a segment of a person's life and existence. It is a physical expression, in part, of a person's spirituality. Thus, it suffices to say that 'I express my spirituality through my religious belief.' This is more like the relationship that exists between a 'whole' and a 'part.' The 'whole' is greater than the 'part.' That is, 'religiosity' portends a set of belief systems or religious practices; direct reference to organized faith group or identification; a measure of such religious practice couched in labels such as "pious," "faithful or devoted," "sanctimonious," "devout" etc. It is, in part, an outward demonstration of one's spirituality, revealing "where" and "how" one practices his/her faith. Spirituality, in a nutshell, is "who" you are and "what" you do in harmony with your true being. For this reason, Wintz and Cooper assert that, "everyone is a spiritual being," while they also hold that, "not everyone is religious." In sum, the followings are the key points to remember about spirituality, especially as it relates to providing such care in a health care environment:

- ◈ Religion is not the same as spirituality.

- It's a melding of connectedness – with a higher power, with others, and with the surrounding world – as a person seeks meaning into life's journey.

- It's at the core of a person's being and usually is conceptualized as a "higher" experience or a transcendence of oneself.

- Such an experience involves a perception of a personal relationship with a supreme being, such as God.

- It encompasses feelings and thoughts that bring meaning and purpose to human existence or to one's life journey.

- Spirituality is known and experienced in relationships: Horizontal (Humans, Nature & Environment); Vertical (God, Transcendent Being)[9]

In relation to serving the needs of patients, families, and hospital staff, spiritual care is:

- Giving professional attention to the subjective spiritual and religious worlds of the care receiver.

- Such individual or subjective worlds include perceptions, assumptions, feelings, and beliefs that connect the individual to the Divine or the Transcendent Being while such subjective relationship is used to interpret real life situations or story such as successes, adversities, illness, hospitalization, death, and life after death.

Pastoral Care Differentiated

"What is the difference between pastoral care and spiritual care? A conference attendee asked at a conference hosted by the United States Navy Bureau of Medicine and Surgery in partnership with the Smithsonian Institution in Washington, D.C. The conference was dubbed: "Wounded Warrior Care: Rediscovery of the meaning of healthcare in America today" in April, 2011. It drew a wide range of healthcare providers, but more importantly, it drew vast majority of hospital chaplains working in the Washington, DC metropolitan area. The panel as well as some participants wrestled with the question until it was laid to rest without succinct consensus. What a legitimate question! At the end of the intellectual wrestling, there seemed not to be a clear-cut answer to the question. I wondered if the questioner might have been disappointed, thinking that he would resolve the "puzzle" easily in the gathering of such a large and experienced group of chaplains and intellectuals. Is it that the line of distinction is blurred? Or, are they – pastoral care and spiritual care – actually the same? Perhaps, it's just a matter of semantics? For whatever it is, the seeming "confusion" and lack of clarity that pervaded the conference room is symptomatic of what an average chaplain or pastor faces when called upon to minister to the needs of the sick. Without much ado, let's cut to the chase! What is pastoral care?

In its general understanding, pastoral care refers to the ministries usually performed by ordained pastors. Etymologically, "pastoral" roots in Middle English, Old French, and Latin *pastoralis.* It is an adjective for 'pastor' which translates 'shepherd' (thefreedictionary.com). A pastor is seen as a shepherd or porter of God's flock. This is referenced in the words of St. Peter: "Be shepherds of God's flock that is under your care, serving as overseers, not because you must, but because you are willing, as God wants you to be… (1 Pet 5:2-3).

Thus "pastoral" is an ecclesiastical (Christianity) term relating to a set of responsibilities, duties or care of a clergy or a priest over a church or a congregation. Pastoral care, therefore, may typically depict services and ministries provided for affiliated members within the confines of the sacred tradition of the Christian group. This may include, but is not limited to, prayers, sacraments, rituals, ministerial presence, biblical counseling, etc. It has become a traditional norm for pastors to be called upon to visit the sick members of their church, sometimes upon individual's request and sometimes based on the discretion of the pastor or the relationship that exists between the pastor and the sick person (or family). That 'pastoral care' is often associated with 'pastor' and his or her vocational duties toward the laity are underscored by literature and authors. For example, John Patton writes: "…pastoral care – a kind of doing that is strongly affected by what the pastor knows and what she is – her presence." Elsewhere, he says: "The pastoral career, whether laity or clergy..."[10]

This reason, perhaps, also underlies Ronald H. Sunderland's brilliant work, entitled "The Dignity of Servanthood in Pastoral Care," tracing the concept of servanthood as a dominant image of ministry in Jewish and Christian traditions. This, according to him, "poses a rich source of material from which to address the theme of human dignity from the perspective of pastoral care." He surmised: "The biblical concept of servanthood, which defines the nature of the pastoral relationship and dignifies the personhood of the care recipient, suggests an approach to the issues of vulnerability of both giver and receiver of care..." Commenting on "Pastoral Care of Dying,' K.C. Brownstone writes: "The caring pastor is a symbol of religious faith."[11]

The limited connotation of the word 'pastor' or 'pastoral' to a particular segment of religious tradition makes its usage for the services provided for hospitalized patients religiously insensitive. Is it appropriate to say that a chaplain provides pastoral care for a Muslim patient? How about a Hindu, a Buddhist, a Jewish, a Quaker..? It is not unusual to find hospitals affiliated to religious institutions tag their department's services as "Pastoral Care Department" while private hospitals tend to prefer "Spiritual Care Department." Some hospitals, however, prefer to combine the two descriptive services – "Pastoral / Spiritual Care Department." The services provided to care-seekers, regardless of the descriptive name chosen - pastoral or spiritual - by these hospitals – or whether they're private or religiously affiliated – may be similar or even the same. The nomenclature, sometimes, is chosen in order to accommodate all and to be religiously inclusive and sensitive.

However, the subtle but profound difference between the two concepts places some limited understanding and non-inclusive disposition toward "pastoral care." Suffice it to say that interfaith is better promoted when an interfaith concept, "Spiritual Care," is used to denote the noble services provided for care seekers without being offensive or insensitive to their religious beliefs. 'Spiritual care' is more inclusive while 'pastoral care' is restrictive in its practical application, especially in healthcare. Albeit, not until the Enlightenment of the 18th century, did religions generally include physical healing in their ministry to whole people![12]

Finally, it is imperative to remember that not all chaplains, working in hospitals, are pastors. It suffices to have religious affiliation and be recognized or endorsed as such. How, then, do we speak of what such a brilliant and dedicated chaplain provides outside the tenets of a pastor's duties? The idea of 'wholeness' then underscores a chaplain's service and ministry. Some Christian groups such as the Quakers neither ordain nor engage in ministerial roles; yet, they believe in care for the sick.

Spiritual Care in the Desert of Illness
-The Chaplain

At the center of a trained chaplain's professional engagement is the art of listening. Rachel Naomi Remen, a Medical Doctor, describes the art of listening succinctly in her book, Kitchen Table Wisdom, when she says: "Listening is the oldest and perhaps the most powerful tool of healing. It is often through the quality of our listening and not the wisdom of our words that we are able to effect the most profound changes in the people around us. When we listen, we offer with our attention an opportunity for wholeness. Our listening creates sanctuary for the homeless parts within the other person."[13] Contextually, the work of providing spiritual care for a care seeker is majorly provided by the institution's chaplains, but also, by community clergies, who are, by geographical proximity, are connected to the care institution, or family clergies. Regardless of the professional category, at the heart of the ministry to the sick is an invaluable listening presence of the spiritual care provider, aimed at bringing holistic healing or "wholeness" as Dr. Remen rightly calls it. In fact, as she surmises, "listening creates a holy silence."[14]

Spiritual Assessment

Performing spiritual assessment is a great in-road to providing targeted spiritual or pastoral care that meets the patient's spiritual or pastoral needs. This spiritual assessment must be differentiated from the Assessment Tools (Triggers for a Spiritual Care consult) later discussed in chapter six. The spiritual assessment here discussed has been developed essentially for the professional use of chaplains and chaplains-in-training to determine the spiritual needs of the care-receiver for the purpose of intentionally addressing such needs and to achieving effective pastoral/spiritual care outcomes. The assessment tool discussed in chapter six is a new initiative developed for the professional use of clinicians and other care team in determining the patient's indirect request for a chaplain. The awareness tool helps to create deeper understanding of the chaplain's roles in the care team as well as chaplain's services to the hospital community. Although suffice to say that chaplains also benefit from the assessment tool as it enhances the knowledge of their professional duties, along with other care team, in a health care environment.

Experts have offered different spiritual assessment tools, both for the chaplain's use, and also for clinicians who are able to incorporate spiritual care into their medical practice. For the purpose of this book, we shall highlight two spiritual assessment tools.

- ◈ FICA (Faith; Importance & Influence; Community; and, Address or Application)
- ◈ SPIRIT (Spiritual belief system; Personal spirituality; Integration with a spiritual community; Ritualized practice and restrictions; Implications for medical care; and, Terminal event planning)

Support for patients and families

Routinely and as will be discussed under the 'Triggers for a spiritual care consult,' chaplains are vital compassionate support for patients as well as their family members, as they are daily confronted with the challenges of hospitalization and aridity of living in the desert of new medical diagnosis and/or poor prognosis. Such supports would include trauma code, cardio-pulmonary resuscitation (CPR) code, decision-oriented family meetings, End of life conversations, supporting grieving families or staff through grief counseling & bereavement care.

Dispensation of the Holy Sacraments

This applies to churches or faith traditions that support sacramental ordination. If ordained or authorized by your faith tradition, provide sacraments (Baptism, Anointing of the sick and/or Last Rites, Reconciliation, or even sacrament of matrimony, etc). Also the chaplain may fulfill specific assistance or prayers as pastorally needed and requested. Chaplains and clinicians should understand that the hospital is an "extraordinary" place of administering these sacraments of faith. That is, hospitalization period should not be typically used either by patients or by family members to accomplish the necessity of sacrament conferment if there is no danger of death (end-of-life). The "extraordinary" religious nature of the hospital is thus invoked for the purposes mentioned above when death is imminent. Extra caution should also be taken by zealous hospital staff to refrain from infant baptism unless one of the two parents or reliable family member expressly gives consent. Cases abound in which children of non-Christian faith were baptized and thus leading to a legal suit against such hospitals. This will be elaborated in Chapter Eight – Christian Tradition and Death & Dying.

Ensuring the spiritual wellbeing of the Clinical Care providers

It is very important to support the care providers in ensuring their wellbeing and wholeness, knowing that their holistic wellness contributes to the safety of the patients entrusted to their care. Why care for the clinicians? This will be fully explored in chapter six.

The Holistic Approach of the Chaplain's Service

Professional Chaplains, as well as community clergy or spiritual or pastoral care providers, have the responsibility to provide care for the **totality** of the human person, beginning with the gift of non-judgmental listening presence. Focusing on the human person in entirety enhances holistic care approach. This approach, initiated and deepened in a non-judgmental listening presence, the chaplain may be able to journey with the patient or the care receiver toward holism in addressing some of the following pastoral or spiritual concerns:

❖ **Resultant Situational Outcome**

What result is the present *situation or experience* yielding? – Positive and growth. That is, whether or not the patient is able to make meaning out of the illness or hospitalization experience, which may lead to the union of body, soul and spirit. It may as well be yielding negative outcome. That is, reduction or regression which results in disunity in the human person, leading to discouragement or despair or depression.

❖ **Resultant Spiritual Outcome**

How are the illness and the entire hospitalization experience affecting the life or spiritual journey or the relationship between the patient and his or her faith? Is he mad at God, so much so that he does not want to talk about God or anything pertaining to "faith?" Or, do you still see the green light of hope and faith as you sit to ponder with her the medical journey thus far? What are you listening for? What spiritual concepts and expressions are repeatedly said by the patient? I once visited a patient, sometime in 2007, which left me with quite an experience to remember. I was in my visible clerical attire, a clergy shirt, aka, clerical shirt. My pastoral task for the day was to visit catholic patients in the assigned units. On meeting patient X, I introduced myself, as I typically do, or as required by the professional protocol of hospital chaplaincy. I had hardly finished the introduction when the patient said, "Don't even bother to talk to be about God… don't! Which God will be a good God and see me lying here on this sick bed? I have been a good catholic all my life…I just don't wanna hear about…" Does this sound like someone experiencing a deep sense of abandonment by God?

❖ **Resultant Experiential Interpretation**

What interpretation is the patient, as you sit and listen, giving to his or her experience in the here and now? How does the individual see or interpret sickness/illness? Is it considered as adversity resulting from wrong deeds? That is, 'am I paying for my sins?' Or, does the individual's spirituality accommodates pain, suffering, illness, sickness and discomforts as part of human mortal nature? Does he/she even want to talk or hear about God? Perhaps, sickness is perceived as a sign of God's abandonment, or a rejection, or Divine injustice?

◆ **Resultant *First-thing-First* Principle**

Attentive listening can help identify the most pressing of all needs besetting the care receiver. Care providers, often time, miss what tops the list of concerns of the patient, especially in the *here-and-now* due to inattentive listening or simply inadvertently presumes what the patient seems to need at that point in time. In some cases, if not many, spiritual care providers, as good listeners, have been the bridges that convey the dearest concern from the patient to the care personnel whose task is it to meet such a need. Attentive listening, hence, will help to identify such concern as: 'What becomes top priority to the patient *here and now?*' It could well be that, the unexpected hospitalization did not allow Ms. Y to put her house in order prior to calling EMS (Emergency Medical Services) or 911. Perhaps, Mr. Z seems worried to death about what might happen to his wife – his companion and friend for the past 55 years. Who knows, the patient was deeply concerned about his dog that was, unfortunately, "abandoned" to no one's care due to medical emergency that led Mr. Z to the ER (Emergency Room)! Healthcare providers might be quick to assume for their patients what their priorities "should" be or "might" be at a given time. However, conversations with patients have shown that we often assume wrongly. We'd thought that a patient would be concerned, primarily, about their health issues or how the individual is dealing with the new diagnosis. Often, what preoccupies the patient's mind is outside the walls of the hospital.

For example, I once was consulted for an oncology patient, Mr. Right. The clinical staff was concerned that "he seemed depressed because of his cancer diagnosis... and so would need someone to "cheer" him up. That was a sincere concern for her patient! Mr. Right sat at the edge of his hospital bed when I visited. He was receptive to a spiritual care visit. Following our exchange of pleasantries, I asked him, 'What's going on, Mr. Right? You seem to be down...' He said: "Yeah, I'm sad because I didn't plan to stay here for five days. I came to the ER (Emergency Room)...hoping that I'll go home the same day. I had put out my girlfriend because we had a disagreement, I locked the house and came to the hospital with the house key...Now that I've been here for the past five days, and I'm worried about her. She may not have a place to stay." That was an issue of great concern for Mr. Right! Everything else may have to wait until he was able to process the feelings and figure out how to ensure the safety of his girlfriend so as to free his conscience from the "guilt" should any unfortunate incident befall her.

❖ Resultant Impact of Hospitalization on the Patient's Family

The amount of weight that hospitalization, or critical illness, can place on family members can sometimes be unimaginable. Studies have shown that patients' family members and loved ones also share in the burden of hospitalization or the challenges that the critical illness may be posing. It is crucial to mention that the illness can impact the patient's family positively or negatively. In many instances, this has impacted families negatively, placing weights of inconvenience, financial strains, emotional burdens, psychological defeats, etc. on close-knit families. For example, on his hospital bed, Mr. Z thinks about so many realities starring at him in the face. The least of these realities might be the next medication that the nurse will soon come to administer, or the next scheduled procedure for which the transporter is almost at the door to wheel him. He might be now confronted with the reality of his broken family, such as his estranged children with whom he has not been in communication for several years or other troubled family dynamics. 'What happens if I don't come out of this procedure?' he might ask himself. Or, Mr. Paulson has been estranged from his own siblings since their mom died twenty years earlier. He is now confronted with his own mortality and grapples with the possible irreconcilable differences with his brothers and sisters. The thought of possible failure to reconcile tortures him more than the surgeon's knife. His sleepless nights have little to do with current hospitalization but more to do with the tension ravaging his family. On a happier note, I once visited a grandma who had been referred for spiritual care consult because she was said to be "withdrawn and un-engaging." During my spiritual care conversation, grandma was apparently sad because she would miss her granddaughter's wedding coming up in the next week and a half. There was not the slightest indication that she would be ready for discharge before the wedding date. The thought of missing her granddaughter's wedding, which she raised, seemed excruciating. She expressed her sadness in tears as I sat to process the feelings with her. 'Why would God allow this to happen?' was one of the many rhetorical questions we both addressed.

◈ Resultant Impact of the Health Condition on the Patient's worldview

Experiences, challenges, and life situation have been known to be concrete elements that can shape a person's worldview. This worldview is open to reevaluation and consequently to change or redefinition, according to the person's interpretation of his or her current challenges and trials. The resultant outcome of the desert experience, during hospitalization or confronted by new critical health diagnosis, can adversely change the patient's worldview. A spiritual care provider may hear phrases such as, "…it's not fair…this life is just not fair…" "…I don't deserve this…" "…she's been a good person…she doesn't deserve this…" Worldview, in this case, may include how the patient sees life and mortality – transient or intransient.

Each of the cases discussed above exemplify the need for spiritual care. Fowler and Peterson capture the essence of spirituality or spiritual care when they write: "Spirituality is the way in which a person understands and lives life in view of her or his ultimate meaning, beliefs, and values… It integrates, unifies, and vivifies the whole of a person's narrative or story, embeds his or her core identity, establishes the fundamental basis for the individual's relationship with others and with society, includes a sense of the transcendent, and is the interpretive lens through which the person sees the world. It is the basis for community for it is in spirituality that we experience our co-participation in the shared human condition."[15] Premised on these principles of "integration," "unification," and "vivification" of the whole human person, as succinctly put by Fowler and Peterson, it is reasonable to describe the roles of chaplains as a ministry of **Care and Support** that fosters the "interconnectedness with self, others, nature, and God."[16]

Chaplains or other pastoral and spiritual care providers, such as community clergy or faith leaders, are invited to provide spiritual support to the care seeker, bearing the following five effective spiritual and pastoral care elements (ECCCD) in mind:

- ✔ **Empathy** – *'Be concerned.'* Empathy, as correctly expressed by Doehring, involves "two simultaneous and opposite relational skills." They are: "making connection with another person by experiencing what it is like to be that person," and, "maintaining separation from the other person by being aware of one's own feelings and thoughts."[17]

- ✔ **Compassion** – *'Com'* (with) & *'passion'* (to *suffer*). Enter the patient's world with these concepts to rule the visit: sympathy, concern, care, sensitivity, warmth, mercy, leniency, kindness, humanness, tenderness, and love.

- ✔ **Companionship** – Journey with the patient as with a friend on an evening walk.

- ✔ **Care-*without*-judgment** – Do not take charge, control, or ascend the judgment seat. Provide care-without-judgment! Standing by the patient's hospital bed isn't a time to adjudge the patient as "*a good and practicing*" Christian or…

- ✔ **Do not try "*to-fix*"** – The care-seeker isn't a piece of broken equipment to be fixed!

It is pertinent for a chaplain to be aware that each encounter with a patient or patient's family or staff portends a "two-way" experience of "giving-and-receiving." The chaplain does not stand to teach the "recipient" of what is right or wrong. The sacred space provided by the patient or any other "recipient" is never turned into a classroom nor does the chaplain have to open solution manuals, trying to fix what he or she feels is broken. Hence, it is important for a chaplain to honor the sacred space of the patient or whoever owns the space (families or staff) and consider such encounter as an invaluable privilege to share the person's life and story. When a chaplain feels that s/he is there to "give," and that the other person "must receive" whatever s/he has to offer, the chaplain, then, might unconsciously control and dominate the conversation, might likely do more talking than listening thereby missing salient but significant points in the moment, might struggle to proffer "solutions" where not needed, and might end up grossly missing the mark. Doehring also discusses the problem of "fusion" in her book "The Practice of Pastoral Care" (2006), which may be a "red flag" or an indicator of when a chaplain "takes over" a spiritual or pastoral care conversation. "Fusion," she writes, occurs "when caregivers become too immersed in the care-seeker's experience." That is, "over-identifying with a care-seeker," she expatiates, "can make it difficult for a caregiver to be aware of her [his] own feelings and at the same time monitor what is happening in the relationship." In brief, as we listen to care-seekers' stories and empathize, we, as chaplains, are warned not to become "over-involved in helping care-seekers."[18]

More often than not, a patient simply needs someone to listen to their stories, validate their concerns and pains, put some smiles on their faces amidst unpleasant realities of life, etc. Since it is common knowledge that doctors or nurses rarely have enough time to sit with a patient, considering the many patients on their care list, chaplains may then be a wonderful bridge to offer that which is lacking in the necessary care of care-seekers. The idea of a chaplain as a bridge will be further elucidated later in the book. Chaplains are trained to be a listening presence. It can be psychologically healing when someone is listened to. On the other hand, it can be traumatizing when one's feelings are neglected, not listened to or a voice being unheard.

Although it is generally acceptable to talk about providing spiritual care through other disciplines in the healthcare – doctors, nurses, etc, it is more appropriate that the spiritual needs of the patients or family members or staff are handled by the chaplains since they are professionally trained to provide such noble services. This notion is better captured by Babler: "Although many members of the healthcare team may address patient's spiritual needs, chaplains are typically the main purveyors of spiritual care in healthcare settings."[19]

Final Thoughts…

The following tips are suggestions and/or reminders for all pastoral and spiritual care ministers. They are by no means exhaustive, but they can serve as useful tools that are often destined to yielding positive pastoral outcomes.

- Be the ***gentle presence of God or the Holy One*** amidst the stormy sea of life confronting the patient or family or any other care-seeker.

- Be ***creative and allow for flexibility*** as each patient, family or care-seeker is unique – avoid stereotypes, associations of events / stories, etc. Remember that no two stories are exactly the same, not even for identical twins.

- Be a ***listening presence***. Listen more, talk less! A listening ear discerns more, a discerning mind offers words of wisdom and healing! Dr. Remen shared her initial misconception about 'listening': "…I had been taught since I was very young. I thought people listened only because they were too timid to speak or did not know the answer."[20] As a pastoral care provider, what is your own perception or struggle around listening ability during your pastoral visits to the sick?

- Not all visits or encounters ***must end with prayer***. Discern where and when prayer is appropriate. Prayer, sometimes, could be a sign of a chaplain's discomfort, embarking on "quick exit" aka "chaplain-on-the-run." Prayer is ***one*** important aspect of what we do as chaplains. Staying in the moment while you offer the precious gift of your comforting presence can soothe like alabaster oil. Also, remember that '*doing an act of charity*' to respond to the immediate needs of the patient or family would be 'prayer' itself. This is what St. Thomas Aquinas would describe as a corporeal act of charity.

- Remember to develop spiritual/pastoral relationship.

- If you have ***no*** word to say, silence can be golden – it can be more comforting! "A loving silence often has far more power to heal and to connect than the most well intentioned words."[21]

Chapter Two

The Desert of Illness[22]

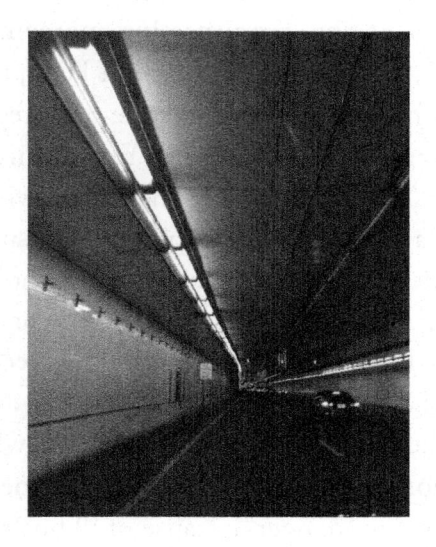

The tunnel can be long, real long, and seemingly unending! The tunnel of the desert can often time be dark and really scary, especially when one finds oneself there unexpectedly. The long and seemingly unending dark tunnel is often lonely.

In this chapter, we shall identify the "Desert of illness," attempt to understand the challenges of life in the Desert, discuss and know the risk factors for 'Spiritual Distress,' highlight care providers' response to 'Spiritual Distress,' and finally, initiate an appeal that will focus on "where do we go from here: From the Desert to Home: A call to Community Clergy."

The Desert Identified

Vacationers could plan and choose their vacation sites and cities. Homeowners or renters could choose preferred communities, cities, or even states whenever they so desire to relocate. These are ample opportunities imbued with great flexibilities in the choice making. Hence, a vacation dream can be realized, a dream home and neighborhood can translate into reality! However, the human prerogative of choice is sometimes hard-hit and could face the unexpected reality that challenges the power to choose – sometimes there is inability to choose due to an emergent health situation, leaving neither time nor the luxury of choice. The clock ticks, the countdown begins, every passing moment is more precious than ever! And then, just as Jesus told Simon Peter, his disciple, "…you will stretch out your hands, and someone else will dress you and lead you where you do not want to go" (Jn 21: 18). You're conscripted to a desert you'd rather not go. To cut straight to the chase, 'who wants to be in a hospital?' Although a synonym for 'hospital' would suggest 'rest home,' I bet everyone would rather rest in their individual homes rather than in a hospital! And yet, a hospital can easily become or be referred to as a 'community'. It is in this sense that although it is a necessary community; yet, it falls under the less preferred community. It is a community where healing and cure takes place; yet, aside from those who earn their daily living there, it is not a community where someone looks forward to visiting other than one in "danger" because of ill health.

Understanding the Challenges of Hospitalization

Life is full of challenges, numerous and diverse. It is even more so with hospitalization experience! In discussing some notable challenges associated with hospitalization, the four basic assumptions about hospital environment[23] will be used as the discussion lens. These are: Experiencing crisis, Change, Spiritual growth and/or emotional/spiritual scars, and, Healing.

Louis Nieuwenhuizen, in the article, *"Spiritual Care Illustrated: Creating a Shared Language,"*[24] discussed the "Four Basic Assumptions about Hospital Ministry." I consider these "Four Basic Assumptions" to be crucial, not only for chaplains or pastoral/spiritual care providers, but even for family members of the hospitalized to understand. I'd like to refer to these "Basic Assumptions" as unavoidable 'Realities' as well as 'Expectations' of those confined to hospital beds or confronted with the reality of human mortality or those who might simply become "needy" of spiritual help as a result of other life realities outside the hospital. These Four *Must-Know* realities and expectations, described as "Basic Assumptions" by Nieuwenhuizen, are: experiencing crisis, change, spiritual growth and/or emotional/spiritual scars, and, healing. As it applies to our focus in this book, we shall now discuss each of these four adapted essential elements, an understanding of which would tremendously enhance care providers' perceptions and services to care receivers.

Experiencing Crisis

Experts and researchers have identified and established logical correlations between hospitalization and stress or anxiety experienced by patients.[25] It is appropriate, says Nieuwenhuizen, to interpret the "stress and anxiety" experienced in the course of hospitalization as symptomatic of "experiencing a crisis." Van Pelt, succinctly defines crisis as "a time when a certain situation overpowers (or strains) that individual's coping mechanisms." Hospitalization could be like a stormy sea for some patients. As such, the sea of their lives would seem to face turbulent waves. While their ship is sailing on a stormy sea, faith is challenged and hope is waning. Daily routines and regimens are either altered or completely suspended. An hour spent in the confinement of hospitalization would seem like five hours in the comfort of one's home. Everything sounds the same, and all you have is hospital regimens which remind you of your powerlessness and limited control over the events of every hour. It is quite understandable if a patient gets frustrated because of "unavoidable" issues such as temporary "incarceration," inability to sleep uninterruptedly, limited privacy, tasteless hospital food, overtime with television, corridor noise, and so on. These are nothing but crisis-inducing agents, not even including the crisis of medical diagnosis that the patient stands to face.

Conducting a research survey on "Impact of hospitalization on patients and families," Subramanina, for T.B. Research Center, I.C.M.R.

Madras states: "Hospitalization, especially for chronic diseases, can have a number of varied effects upon a patient and his or her family members. Those effects were assessed among a sample of patients seen at Tuberculosis Research Center, Chennai. Two hundred consecutive patients of a mean age of 23.7 years upon admission with tuberculosis of the spine were considered for study. The patients were aged 18 months to 60 years. There were 130 patients hospitalized, of whom 63 belonged to the operated category. Fifty-four patients were in the hospital for 4-5 months, 54 for 6 months, and 22 for more than 9 months to a maximum duration of 18 months. A number of personal and other problems related to hospitalization are listed. Noted by 84% of hospitalized patients, financial difficulties comprised by far the most often noted problem. Also 34% noted home sickness, 20% boredom, 18% an effect upon household responsibilities, and 17% an effect upon a household member's education" (Indian J Public Health, 1998).

This is a valuable backdrop that chaplains and clinicians will have to constantly remember as they provide the needed care and support for hospitalized patients or caregivers. According to a more recent survey, 73.2% of patients surveyed indicate that their hospitalization experience is "significantly or totally overwhelming."[26] This, for Van Pelt, would constitute a crisis experience. It must be said that the vast majority of hospitalized patients would rather not be there if they'd had a choice. That is, the fact that many or most patients are unavoidably in the hospital, against their wish and comfort, signals "crisis experience." The question for a visiting care-provider (physician, nurse, chaplain, social worker, dietician, etc.), then, is 'How do I help to reduce the prevailing stress?' Or, for the chaplain, 'How do I process this "crisis experience" with the patient?' Or, 'How do I journey with the patient to recognize and accept the reality of life in the here and now?' Realizing that the patient's story has changed from, perhaps, "I have never been sick all of my life," to "… now you are at MedStar Washington Hospital Center because you are sick." Based on the outcomes of this research, these hints and concerns will be very helpful for care-providers to remember, knowing that patients do face different life prevailing situations and contend with the burdens of hospitalization in varied ways such as:

- ❖ Financial burdens:
  - Limited or lack of medical insurance;
  - Affordability of prescribed medications and subsequent mandatory hospital follow-ups;
  - Harassments from never-ending medical bills
  - No-work-no-pay syndrome;
  - Mortgage(s) and home utility bills;
  - Parental and other social responsibilities, etc
- ❖ Nosocomephobia (fear/phobia of hospital)
- ❖ Loneliness and boredom
- ❖ High level of vulnerability
- ❖ Obstruction to family or other social pre-planned engagements (Family reunion at Thanksgiving, Christmas, New Year, wedding, etc)

Change

For some patients, their first hospitalization begins a life-changing experience. For instance, patients diagnosed with diabetes, benign mass or tumor; trauma resulting from domestic violence (gunshot wound, stabbing, etc.), natural disaster (fire, storm or inclement weather, etc), or for some other plausible reasons. Research has shown that 'change' can seem distinctly unfriendly to humans much more a life-altering change or experience. *Change*, for a patient, may be defined as the inability to revert to preadmission condition. For instance, a newly diagnosed type 2 diabetic patient: a *change* from pre-condition to new condition (diabetic); a *change* from "free" lifestyle (unrestricted food or drink) to controlled daily diet; a *change* from non regimented life to daily monitoring of blood glucose, etc. Or, a cardiac patient placed on a waiting list for a heart transplant and in the interim will have to use a LVAD (Left Ventricular Automatic

Device) device to keep the heart functioning. He or she has to carry the device wherever and whenever. It is a life changing experience, learning to follow some set of stipulations. Or, think of a transplant survivor who will definitely have to maintain precautious regiments and compliance in order to avoid the risk of rejection and post-transplant complications. This is a change that could alter the rhythm of life. According to Carol Kent, such a *change* can be called "a new kind of normal."

Spiritual growth and/or emotional/spiritual scars

That human beings respond to life situations and experiences differently is supported by vast data and research outcomes. The varied responses, without a doubt, will be predicated upon numerous factors including spiritual disposition of the individual. The disposition informs the "hermeneutic" of interpretation or internalization. For some, their hospitalization can be a step upward in reaching closer to God or attaining deeper relationship with the Supreme Being or even rectification of relationships. For some others, getting lost in an unfamiliar desert of sickness and the inability to get numerous questions answered can lead several steps away from God or to fragmentation within the self. Relationship with the Supreme Being can either be strained or completely ruptured. Either for spiritual growth or spiritual regression, a hospitalization experience could become a pathway to a "new" spirituality. For those whose spiritual disposition would interpret their hospitalization experience positively, the story of Job in the Holy Bible is a classic story, for Christians especially, that teaches patience, trust, acceptance, steadfastness, faith, and hope. It is a story of strength for those who resonate with it. Often in spiritual or pastoral conversation, Job's story easily becomes a reference point. In one of his responses to his wife, Job said: "…We accept good things from God; should we not accept evil?" (Job 2:10).

Patients and/or families in this spiritual category are usually receptive to spiritual visits from chaplains, pastors or clergy from their faith communities. They often request regular visits and prayers from spiritual or pastoral care providers. In addition to their psycho-emotional upbeat, they often display calm posture in dealing with the reality of their sickness, and are imbued with patience and resilience. This is not without its ups and downs, good days and bad days. All in all, the individual views "this" (hospitalization or health situation) as a "phase," a "trial," or a "passing storm." When this "storm" eventually passes or the individual is able to accept and make peace with the irreversible health condition, there is the great possibility for spiritual growth. If, on the other hand, a patient or caregiver interprets the pressing situation of hospitalization or health situation negatively, this can lead to overwhelming frustrations, anger, emotional and spiritual distress – all that has been said above in favor of spiritual growth in reverse. Such psycho-emotional disposition is characterized by negative feelings, rejection and/or unreceptiveness to many forms of support – spiritual, social, clinical (if possible), etc. People in this spiritual category often see and interpret their hospitalization or health situation as a sign of God's rejection and abandonment. Their "uprightness" is often contrasted with the "unmerited" hospitalization. Hence, God is perceived as unjust, and their illness as an act of injustice. It is not unusual, therefore, for chaplains to become victims of negative feelings from such patients or family members since chaplains are seen as God's representatives. This is a typical case of transferred aggression – chaplains or spiritual/pastoral care-providers have to answer for God.

Consider one of my experiences. I embarked on my daily routine visits to patients, per the religious census, of my assigned nursing units. The Pastoral Care department of the hospital meets the spiritual needs of patients and families by dividing all nursing units among the chaplains. Hence, I had the responsibility for the spiritual well-being of all patients on my nursing units regardless of their religious affiliations or faith traditions. I stopped by to visit with Ms. Novo. Incidentally, I wore a visible sign that marked me as a Catholic priest – my clerical shirt. Since the patient could see me from the entrance door, she motioned to me (without words) to turn around and leave. I said, "Thank you, ma'am" and I exited the room.

A chaplain colleague once shared with me that he had stopped by to visit one of his patients on three separate occasions but each of the 'stop bys' was greeted with unreceptive behaviors. Clinicians are not, in anyway, left out as recipients of such negative vibes. In fact, they more often than not meet with stonewalls as they try to provide services that will help such patients and/or family members. This could take the form of non-compliance, rejection of medication or medical services, complete or partial shut-downs, etc. This is further discussed in Chapter Six – 'The Triggers for a Spiritual Care Consult'. It is very essential to recognize what underlies a patient's refusal or blatant rejection of services from care providers. Chaplains, unlike other care providers, can use their skill of empathy to see in the very spectacle or eye lens of the patient. Remember, such a patient needs more time, different tone, more of a compassionate presence than informative conversation, a different manner of approach while helping to navigate around other realities of life surrounding the patient including family dynamics, source of support and strength, patient's perspective regarding goals of care, etc.

Healing

All that has been discussed under spiritual growth is very relevant here. It is, presumably, the desire of every patient to be healed. However, it is also true that the healing does occur, but perhaps not as the patient or family expects. An experience well managed cannot but contribute to the healing that the individual desires. It suffices to say that an experience viewed in a positive eye-lens can aid spiritual growth; spiritual growth can, in turn, foster healing. Such healing, within this parameter of understanding, is not restricted but could include physical healing. In other words, the physical healing, as desired by the care-seeker, may not be realistically attainable but its resulting spiritual growth can advance mind and spirit healthiness. It is pertinent to say, however, that patients, depending on the individual's health situation or condition, may further experience any of these spiritual crises ("change"):

- ❖ **Spiritual Disequilibrium**

    Spiritual disequilibrium is the state of inner chaos that results when a patient's most life-threatening illness causes him or her to question previously held assumptions about self-worth or the love and fairness of God.

◆ **Spiritual Need**

A person's spiritual need is considered as any factors necessary to establish and/or maintain one's relationship with God.[27]

◆ **Spiritual Distress**

Spiritual distress is the disruption in the life principle that pervades a person's entire being and that integrates and transcends one's biological and psychosocial nature.

- ◆ Spiritual distress or "*dis-ease*" is a disruption in one's spirit; distress of the human spirit.

- ◆ Such patients who report or indicate – by verbal or nonverbal expressions - that their "spirits are down" or they feel "broken-hearted."

- ◆ Spiritual distress feelings might include a sense of abandonment by God or by others (families or friends); doubts about religious or spiritual beliefs (McLane et al, 1991; O'Brien, 1999; North American Nursing Diagnosis).[28]

- ◆ Searching for meaning of illness as manifested by voicing of "why me?" questions.

- ◆ Quest for purpose in life and self-worth as manifested by such statement as, "Now that I'm confined to a wheelchair, what good am I?"

- ◆ Spiritual distress related to inability to participate in religious practices:

  - Unable to attend mosque or perform ritual Islamic prayers and ablutions as evidenced by the remark, "I feel like I am disobedient to Allah's commands when I can't kneel to prayer like usual."

  - When a Catholic cannot kneel to make sacramental confession as prescribed due to a fragile health condition or some sort of disability.

- A faithful worshipper can no longer gather with community for prayer or community worship and is deeply distressed over the inability.[29]

◈ As published by the National Cancer Institute, 61% of 57 inpatients with advanced cancer receiving end-of-life care in a hospital reported spiritual distress when interviewed by hospital chaplains. Intensity of spiritual distress correlated with self-reports of depression.[30]

◈ **Spiritual pain; Spiritual alienation; Spiritual anxiety, guilt, anger, loss & despair**: "alterations in spiritual integrity."

- Spiritual Pain, most frequent of all, is: An individual's perception of hurt or suffering stemming from feelings of loss or separation from one's God or deity, a sense of personal inadequacy or sinfulness before God, or a pervasive condition of loneliness of spirit.

Possible Hazards from Spiritual Distress[31]

- Blocks to self-love
- Energy-consuming anxiety
- Inability to forgive
- Low self-esteem
- Maturational losses
- Mental illness
- Physical illness
- Physical or psychological stress
- Poor relationships
- Situational losses
- Substance abuse

Consequence of Spiritual Distress[32]

- Altered role performance
- Anticipatory or dysfunctional grieving
- Body image disturbance
- Chronic sorrow
- Death anxiety
- Decisional conflict
- Defensive coping
- Dispiritedness
- Fear
- Hopelessness

- ❖ Impaired social interaction
- ❖ Non-compliance
- ❖ Negative perception to life
- ❖ Risk for loneliness
- ❖ Self-esteem disturbance
- ❖ Social isolation
- ❖ Powerlessness

From the above outlined possible hazards and resulting diagnoses of spiritual distress, it is imperative for care providers, as well as care receivers, to attend their spiritual well-being. It is even more crucial for care providers and caregivers, since their state of mind, disposition and integral wholeness and well-being could affect the quality of care they provide, consciously or unconsciously. It behooves every healthcare community to ensure that safe and quality care for care-seekers are not compromised as a result of spiritual distress. It falls on the leadership of each hospital community to ensure that physicians, nurses, and other care providers are cared for, holistically, in order for their healthy self to engineer healthy care. This will be better elucidated in the following subtitle.

Responding to Spiritual Distress

In responding to spiritual distress, patients, caregivers, and care providers can take the following steps:

Spiritual Health:

- ◆ Harmonious interconnectedness, creative energy and faith in a power greater than oneself are the key attributes of spiritual well-being.
- ◆ Harmonious relationship within the "council" of one's being: body, mind and spirit. That is, maintain wholeness in all dimensions of your beings.
- ◆ Strengthened belief, hope, faith-practice, and inner strength to enhance spiritual quality of life.
- ◆ Manifest endowed inner strength, peace, joy, a sense of purpose

and positive outlook, etc.[33]

Restoration & Rejuvenation:

- ❖ Restoration refers to the ability of a person's spirituality to have a positive influence on the physical aspects of a person.

- ❖ Alterations and changes in disposition or mood portend a need for restoration. Denial and suppression and stonewalling can be very dangerous. On the other hand, accepting and staying in touch with one's humanness can enhance and fortify restoration. It can help to reroute every segment of the person's life that needs to be back on track.

- ❖ Timely restoration enhances progressive and less interrupted rhythm of events in one's life. The earlier the better!

Supporting Your Unique Bridge:

- ❖ Authenticity:

    - ◆ Genuineness and sincerity to self is next to nothing! It is the key that unlocks the door for integral wholeness to the self. That means, not pretending to be a "good" religious patients or unruffled physicians or nurses.

    - ◆ Hospitals remind every human person – patients, clinicians and non-clinicians alike – of human vulnerability and mortality. However, it is **Okay** to show vulnerability in whatever dimension it affects the individual – care-seekers or care providers. Such openness brings help that might be needed.

    - ◆ Holding and supporting the bridge of your life-journey demands authenticity. This begins with unreserved and unpretentious acceptance of one's own uniqueness in all its ramifications, and then, uniqueness in expressing one's feelings. This, sometimes, is hard to encounter in hospitals, especially among physicians. Spiritual distress can be forestalled and restoration can occur without undue delay by dealing authentically with one's feelings and understanding how a particular encounter, for instance, affects your personal or professional rhythms.

- ❖ Be comfortable with your own "wound," your own story, pain, and your own humanness.

- ❖ Bring hope and not judgment to those in the desert of illness and pain. Foster reassurance and allow "to-be."

From the Arid Desert to Home
-A call to Community Faith Leaders for Seamless Care

Where Do We Go From Here? This is a fundamental question that calls for unwavering attention as well as concrete resolution. Often, in the course of my spiritual care visits to patients and families, I have heard the disappointments and the yearnings of patients after their return from the desert of hospitalization to their respective homes. They then suffer pastoral and spiritual "abandonment" from their faith communities. Many ardent Christians who are home-bound would have loved to receive visits from their local pastors for prayers, weekly (at least) Holy Communion, Sacrament of the Sick, counseling, and other spiritual support but they often wait in vain. In fact, some community clergy are unaware of the "sick" members of their flock. Hence, the "weak" members fall outside the pastoral and spiritual radar of the faith community, which disappointedly, makes the home-bounds feel "ostracized" or spiritually forgotten. There is a necessary harmony that exists between mind, body, and spirit. Care for the mind and spirit, as we stated earlier on, cannot but support good physical living. This is why it becomes imperative for community religious leaders to assist the "feeblest" to keep their spiritual connection alive and active, ridding them from a feeling of abandonment and loneliness and spiritual starvation which can "kill" before death itself. Consequently, it is not unusual for the elderly or home-bounds to ask:

- ❖ Who am I to the Community? This is a question of relevance: "In health and sickness; Or, in health ONLY?"

- ❖ It is reasonable to suppose that every member of the flock – sick or healthy – would prefer *Integration* versus *Isolation* from their faith community. That is, pastoral and spiritual care and support should continue seamlessly. Ideally, this is what integration should like:

- ◈ Patient moves from his/her faith Community Desert (hospital Community) and back from the Desert (hospital Community) the faith Community.

- ◈ Statistically, a study of 230 advanced cancer patients in New England and Texas assessed their spiritual needs, according to the National Cancer Institute. It was found that 47% (almost half) reported that their spiritual needs were not being met by their religious communities, while 72% reported that these needs were not supported by the medical system.[34]

When people are beset with the "un-preferred" reality of life by being confined at home or unable to exercise their religious beliefs among a community of believers, this can most certainly feel like another form of the "desert" experience. But, very importantly, these connections enable the home-bounds to continue to experience God's presence and love in the gift of their faith community. Also, such integration can be a source of invaluable strength – emotionally, psychologically, and spiritually – for those "incarcerated" by the frailty of the human body. Hence, it is pastorally and spiritually expedient for Community Clergy, especially for those whose faith traditions encourage such, to look for the "lost" or "ailing" sheep of their faith community in order to make the sheepfold whole. It will be spiritually fulfilling if Community Clergy would:

- ◈ Give them the sense of being remembered through:
  - ◈ Pastoral and spiritual presence for encouragement, support, and prayers.
  - ◈ Sacramental fulfillment by feeding their souls with the food of life they ardently desire.

The seamless *Spiritual wellness* can then be ensured in and out of faith community.

Chapter Three

In the Hallways, In the Waiting Rooms: The Pain of Waiting & Unknown Outcomes

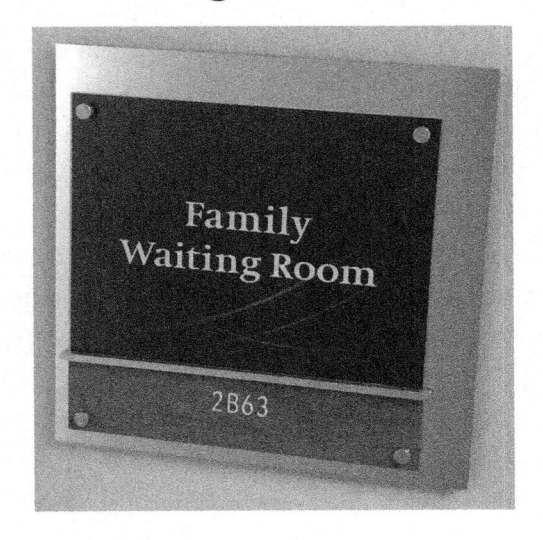

The objectives of this chapter shall include:

- ◈ To understand patients' and families' pain while waiting
- ◈ To understand how clinicians can reduce the waiting time
- ◈ To understand the necessity of timely information

To walk through hallways, to pass by family waiting rooms, or to intentionally look for someone in the waiting areas will be to confront the reality of anxiety and apprehension written boldly on the faces of families and loved ones of patients. Hospital staff, especially anyone in a hospital scrub or wearing hospital ID badge becomes very important during the waiting moment. Approaching gathered or seated family members simply raises the anxiety level as they wonder 'could that be for us?' Eyes are turned toward the hospital staff, expectation is refreshed and ears are itching to hear updates! This is even more true when the patient is in the operating room, popularly called OR, either for a scheduled procedure / surgery or emergency surgery. Even more so when a patient is ambulanced or air-lifted by a reason of trauma – gunshot, stabbing, auto accident, other domestic violence, burn, mass casualties, and so on. One can only imagine the height and weight of anxiety and uncertainty that family and friends of the patient feel.

In the course of my years in hospital chaplaincy work at a level 1 trauma hospital, and especially during my Clinical Pastoral Education (CPE) Residency training program, I have had to stay with families during codes – trauma, yellow, or code heart – to provide the much needed support. The depth of worry written on their faces is indescribable. For a trauma patient, who has just suffered a gunshot wound, for instance, the level of unpredictable outcome is certainly high, especially as perceived by family and friends. Between the arrival of a patient at the trauma center and when the attending physician comes to speak with the family, words cannot describe sufficiently what goes on while families are anxiously waiting. Among other possible reactions are wailings and emotional overload, pacing the hallways or the waiting room, repeated tough questions directed at the non-clinical staff, blames and/or guilt, rejection of offered supportive measures, and so on. While the physicians, nurses and other clinical team members are working tirelessly to "save" the victim, families are pressing to know the outcome, to have their numerous questions answered. One cannot but be sympathetic with families in such a situation; it is human. Think of a cardiac-related problem that necessitated a 911 call and subsequently, an emergent catheterization! Families following behind the ambulance are obviously immersed in the deepest ocean of fear, anxiety and worry. What will the outcome be? A preponderance of rhetorical questions between operating room & waiting room! The weight of hospitalization is not just on the patient in the operating room but also on his/her loved one in the waiting room. It weighs heavily, also, on family members, friends and loved ones who have to spend several hours waiting on the doctor for updates, test results, situational pronouncement, etc. It certainly takes a toll on the spouses who have to sit for several hours and days by the husband's / wife's bedside, watching the monitor and noticing every rhythm of the heart rate – sensitive to the slightest change in the blood pressure counts; etc. Sometimes the caregiver goes without food for several hours as a result of altered rhythm of life or loss of appetite due to the criticalness of the illness.

Think of patients and families waiting in the Emergency Room! You really don't want to think about it, seriously. Neither do you want to experience it! An "Average U.S. ER wait time is 4-plus hours" as claimed by the Health News by United Press International, Inc. (UPI). It was reported, according to Dr. Angela Gardner, president of the American College of Emergency Physicians, who assessed the Press Ganey's Pulse Report 2010, that the report reveals the average length of stay in a U.S. emergency department has increased to 4 hours, 7 minutes.[35] ABC News expressed similar disturbing concern as "ER Wait Times Getting Longer, Survey Says." According to Todd Neale, *MedPage Today* Staff writer, "A patient waiting in a typical emergency department would have time to watch more than four-hour-long episodes of the iconic television show "ER," according to a survey by a national hospital consulting firm."[36] And, CNN Medical Reporter, Sabriya Rice, called the pandemic a nightmare "Don't die waiting in the ER." This is an increase of 31 minutes since 2002, according to the Pulse Report, a hospital consulting firm, that based its survey findings on 1.5 million patients.[37] My experience at a hospital's ER in Maryland, 2005, would support this survey and its subsequent result. I arrived at the hospital at about 5:30pm, called for registration at about 8:50pm, was seen by a physician at my ER bay at some time past 10:00pm. Perhaps that wasn't extraordinarily terrible, right? I was privileged to work with a patient and family in one of the four hospitals I have served as a hospital chaplain. The patient's brother, upon his brother's demise, lamented that they both arrived the hospital's ER at about 7:00pm as a result of intense and persistent pain – sickle cell crisis. He narrated how his brother was crying for help repeatedly but to no avail. Finally, his brother (the patient) encouraged him to go home at about midnight. As he departed the ER, according to him, no medical staff had yet attended to his brother. That is waiting! But maybe this is not even bad enough when compared to a state like Utah, the worst performing state, which had "an increase of 89 minutes in its average time spent in the ER. That brought the total time to 8 hours and 17 minutes, 2 hours and 34 minutes longer than the state with the next longest wait time – Kansas at 5 hours and 43 minutes."[38] Not only are patients subjected to agonizing waiting, but accompanying family members suffer the emotional and psychological torture of seeing their loved ones in agony and excruciating pain within the reach of assistance but no timely help. Listening to patient's frustrations about ER waiting, I have heard some patients remark, "I'd rather fight the pain and discomfort than come to ER…"

As if that was not bad enough, healthcare communities, around the globe, continue to wrestle with the inexplicable pain of waiting. In the United Kingdom, a report indicated that patients' health and treatment could suffer because of waiting-times for x-rays, cardiology tests, ultrasound scans, etc. Statistics show that 15,667 patients waited more than six weeks to undergo a diagnostic procedure in May 2011, a more than fourfold increase on the same month in 2010, when 3,378 did.[39] As typical wait for diagnosis increased from 1.8 weeks to 1.9 weeks (May 2011), in U.K., the implication of this dangerous waiting, invariably, is that the longer waits to access diagnostic tests cause greater anxiety for patients and mean that identification of serious illness such as cancer is delayed.[40] Comparing these stats to the current situation in the United States, a report shows that the United States scored well on physicians' perceptions of how many patients experience long waits for diagnostic tests. A full 57% of physicians in the U.K, and 51% of Canadian physicians reported that their patients experienced long waits for diagnostic tests, compared to only 9% of U.S. physicians who reported the same. The U.K (60%) and Canada (57%) had the highest numbers of persons who had to wait four weeks or more to get to see a specialist physician. In the U.S., only 23% reported a wait of four weeks or more for specialty care.[41]

Possible Consequences of Waiting:

The longer an ill patient has to wait to see a doctor, the greater the chance their sickness will worsen.

- ◈ Wait times places patients' health at risk and costs hospitals, insurers and patients more in resources and dollars.
- ◈ Patients, who give up and walk out, will often get sicker and show up later in worse shape.
- ◈ An Institute of Medicine report on the crisis in U.S. emergency did a study on why wait times are increasing:
  - Doctors overbook patients. Overbooking is usually deliberate because doctors are paid by volume under many health insurance reimbursement systems.
  - Increased demand – the number of patients seeking ER care jumped 26 percent to 114 million in the last few years.
  - Doctor shortages especially in rural areas and certain types of specialties.
  - Hospitals closing the Emergency Room – the number of U.S. emergency departments fell about 12 percent in the last few years. Patients must make a decision to go to a nearby doctor or travel a long distance to find an available emergency room.[42]

One can only imagine what goes on in the minds of the "waiters!" The waiting could result in a patient facing potential serious diagnosis. On the other hand, the waiting could terminate in "non serious" issues. Whichever way it ends, when not properly managed, the final analysis brings a heightened level of uncertainty, worry, anxiety and sleeplessness and loss of appetites and reduced level of enthusiastic spirit about life, etc. I once visited my patient, who was said to be "having a bad day." Her face truly revealed a deeply troubled soul. She shared her disappointment with me, among others, stating that she had gone through several medical tests over the period of 4 -5 days of her hospitalization without receiving a single result. Another test was said to be pending but she showed great reluctance – which was the reason for chaplain's consult. Who wants to keep being subjected to the same or similar examinations repeatedly without result! It is even worse if someone is, unfortunately, admitted over the weekend. But how about during the normal work weeks? It is highly frustrating, not only for patients, but also for families who bear the brunt of inconvenience. It is, nevertheless, sickening for non-clinical care providers such as the chaplains, to be saddled with patients' and families' complaints of the "no-one-is-telling-us-anything" syndrome. Information limbo is a hard place to be! The thought of it, as stated above, could prevent people from seeking a much needed medical attention thereby leading to deterioration of their health condition.

Medicine and technology are gifts to humanity. It is absolutely crucial to remember that, as gifts, they are meant to serve human needs, to reduce human burdens, and, to aid and enhance the quality of human existence. Technology and its use is not meant to replace humanness. Compassion, love, care and humaneness are necessary feelings for humans even in the age of technology. The growth and explosive advancement of modern medicine and technology should not displace these great invaluable attributes – essential factors of care giving. Hence, physicians, nurses and other healthcare workers need to understand how tiring and emotionally draining waiting can be. Considering the waiting instances discussed above, physicians could be mindful of the impact of waiting on their patients and family caregivers in the following ways:

- ❖ If patient is in OR: This concerns both anticipated and non-anticipated long procedures and surgeries – kindly designate a clinical staff member dedicated to keeping family-in-wait updated of the progress. The surgeon can then give a final update when surgery is concluded. Rather than "driving" through a panic tunnel for several hours of the surgery, plus unforeseeable delays, this will help to maintain or reduce the anxiety level.

- ❖ If patient awaits test result: It is very important for patients and/or family caregivers to understand, from the outset, the length of waiting time for the results in question to be available. It doesn't hurt if this is repeated over a period of time, within the waiting period, through the nurse or attending physician. This is necessary because, it is not unusual for patients to fail to fully absorb all information during admission or within the few hours of their hospitalization, especially if serious medical tests are involved. Constant and intermittent reminders will calm patient's anxiety level. Reassure the patient of work-in-progress and assure the individual that he or she has not been forgotten. Also, the patient should be updated if, for any reason, the expected time for the result extends. This can greatly increase and enhance trust between the patient and the care provider.

- ◆ If patient needs multiple tests: It is common that a patient could need several tests within a short period of hospital stay. However, it is essentially important, too, that physicians and other clinical team members present a collaborative team work at all times during the patient-physician encounter. This is facilitated when a visiting physician references previous clinical conversations with patient and/or family, indirectly informing the patient and caregivers that "I (the physician) have read your chart, and that I'm working in collaboration with others for the purpose of seamless holistic care." It can be annoying, frustrating and somehow disgusting when a doctor discusses with a patient or family member the purpose of proceeding on a "required test" without knowing that another doctor has been in the room a few hours prior to inform the patient to the contrary. This was a scenario during a patient's visit. And the doctor said: "Oh, I didn't know that he saw you already…I've not checked the chart…Ok, let me get back to you…" For the purpose of trust and confidence in healthcare system, I, as a patient, would not want to experience "disjointed" or fragmented service. This, surely, could check excessive medical tests occurring in many hospitals, thereby saving the nation some health-related costs.

Chapter Four

The Desert Community
Home of Diversity & Community of All Faiths

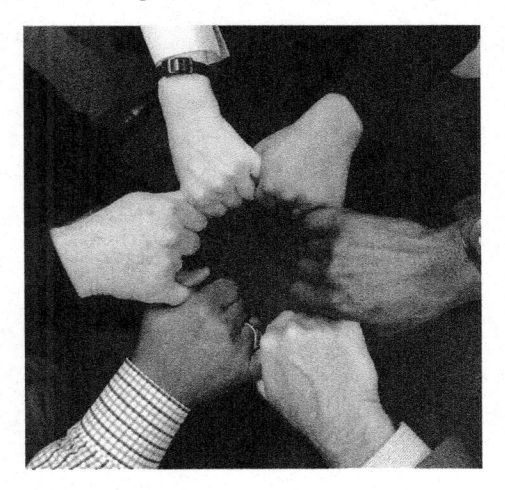

In this Chapter, we shall be able to achieve the following:

- Understand the Ambivalence of "All faiths" (Multi-faith)
- Understand how to provide Spiritual Care without prejudice to others' faith
- Facilitate Community Worship for 'All Faiths – some Topics

The Ambivalence of "All Faiths" in a Hospital Community

"Pluralism, Diversity, Liberalism: Words of Panic or Care?"[43] This was the topic for the Presidential Address delivered by David C. Johnson at the APC Conference Member Recognition Luncheon (June 23, 2012).

The relevance of his topic and of the subsequent conversation intended in this chapter cannot be overemphasized. It is so intriguing to know that the feelings and experience cuts across the world of Spiritual / Pastoral Care providers, so much that it deserved "red carpet" conversation among reputable chaplains. I cannot agree more with Johnson to say that "Within APC [ACPE, NACC, NJC, etc] we have our own nomenclature and buzzwords." Pushing further, he states: "In the APC statements of vision and values, I found these buzzwords:

- Multi-faith [Interfaith] and multicultural professional competency
- Dignity and worth of all persons
- Inclusivity and diversity
- Justice and equality for all"

These "buzzwords" are very prominent in the curriculum of CPE (Clinical Pastoral Education), at least in the two CPE centers where I had my training as a professional chaplain. They are concepts that CPE students and their supervisors often "throw" around either during group sections (IPR, Verbatim, Didactics, etc) or Individual Supervision (IS). That is, the "buzzwords" or concepts are often discussed wherever spiritual or pastoral care involved. However, it feels as if the more often it is talked about, the farther the conversant tend to move away from it! David Johnson rhetorically asked: "Are these buzzwords found in our vision and values statements words of panic or care to you?"

For students who go through the professional training – (CPE) – of providing spiritual care to care-seekers, the above concepts will not be strange as the curriculum is designed to encourage students to step outside the bounds and confines of their individual faith tradition, learn and provide worship services that will be interfaith-oriented. Among other aspects of the CPE curriculum that could possibly pose a challenge to students in training, planning and leading an interfaith worship is certain to take a prominent slot. Its difficulty, it seems, resides not in the didactic or group discussion, but in its planning and execution. Hence, one might be correct to say, "It is easier said than done!" In fact, David Johnson captured the reality of the seeming upheaval faced by spiritual / pastoral care providers when he said: "It is easy to throw them around as concepts until suddenly 'progress' pushes us past our 'traditional' comfort zone. At that point, these words move from a place of care to one of panic."

I recall how difficult it was for me to lead my first interfaith service as a CPE intern in 2005. To say that it was an upheaval would only be for the lack of better expression. You may begin to understand the height of the mountain I had to climb when, as someone born into Catholicism, that's all I have ever known throughout my 34years – to that point – not just as a catholic Christian but as an ordained Roman Catholic priest. I had to lead an assembly comprised of Baptists, Methodists, Unitarians (peer group), and other possible faith traditions that might be in attendance. It seemed beyond my wildest imagination. I was like a fish out of water! Planning the service bulletin was not as difficult as sharing the message. I was oscillating between speaking out of conviction as my faith and catholic theology taught me and being mindful of other faiths and theologies present in the gathering. That is, I struggled to maintain the balance between truthfulness to my faith tradition and respecting others' religious boundaries. It was not an easy task! I needed to affirm without condemnation. I needed to witness without denial. I needed sincerity without falsehood or pretence. Bearing all these in mind, I knew that it wasn't appropriate for me to share the message ("preach") as if I were preaching to a catholic congregation. Images and concepts would be totally out of place. For example, upholding the common early Christian acclamation: "…and every tongue confess that Jesus Christ is Lord, to the glory of God the Father" (Phil 2: 11). Or, about salvation: "For by grace you have been saved through faith…" (Eph 2: 8). Elsewhere, "…that through faith in Jesus Christ the promise might be given to those who believe" (Gal 3: 22); and about the resurrection: "…through him [Jesus] believe in God who raised him [Jesus] from the dead and gave him [Jesus] glory, so that your faith and hope are in God" (1 Pet 1:21). This also dovetailed to prayer formats. As we shall see later in this chapter, some graduates of the CPE program heaved a great sigh of relief – at exit interviews – as they described their struggles with conducting interfaith worship service. Some admit, 'it definitely my growing edges'.

Another experience readily came to mind. I wore double hats as a CPE Resident: first, as a Catholic Priest/Chaplain serving MedStar Washington Hospital Center; MedStar National Rehabilitation Hospital; and, Children's National Medical Center. Also, I was a CPE student (Resident). On a fateful Sunday, I had the pastoral obligation to celebrate Mass for the Catholic patients in the Rehabilitation hospital at 10:00am and then, since I was scheduled as on-call chaplain, I was also responsible to conduct an interfaith service for other patients in the rehab at 11:00am. Enter into my shoes and use your wide imagination!

As I looked up and exclaimed, "…From where will my help come?" (Ps 121: 1) so did my peer group as each student took turns planning and leading the service. As if religious expressions were not enough trouble, then I had to be mindful of language in view of inclusivity.

It is absolutely crucial to say that, whatever perception a spiritual or pastoral care provider might have in view of 'interfaith' or 'multi-faith' or 'diversity' or 'inclusivity' etc, or the difficulty entailed in leading such a "mixed" audience or congregation, it is indisputable that the hospital community is a conglomeration of all possible faiths under the sky. In defining our territory of coverage, chaplains' service will include patients, families, all care providers employed by the hospital or the care facility irrespective of faith traditions or religious affiliations. Even at religiously-owned hospitals or care facilities, freedom of religion and association is a right of every citizen, protected by the nation's Constitution. Hence, not only does this unique right have to be respected, but no care-seeker can be denied receiving faith-specific spiritual or pastoral care in the course of hospitalization. Sometimes, it is easier to accept the diversity of the hospital community *only* in view of 'multicultural' backgrounds. But, it should be within our purview, also, that 'diversity' dovetails into multiple-religion's presence within the establishment. As a hospital chaplain, therefore, it is pertinent to ask: "How do I react whenever I hear or use the concept 'interfaith' or 'multi-faith'?" Or, "What does it invoke in me – panic or care, acceptance or judgment?"

Hans Küng, Swiss Catholic Priest and Professor of Ecumenical

Theology, captured the essence and the necessity of interfaith during a talk entitled *"The World's Religions: Common Ethical Values"*: "There will be no peace among the nations without peace among the religions. There will be no peace among the religions without dialogue among the religions."[44]

According to the Constitution of Interfaith International, religion advocates respect for human rights and freedom of expression. It fosters peace, tolerance and co-existence for all the people of the world. Also, it promotes respect for individuals, their beliefs and faiths, mutual regard for all religious practices and their freedom of expression. It is projected as instruments of the promotion of human rights.[45]

World's Religion, according to the salient but profound points from the Interfaith International, are meant to be an instrument of respect for human rights expressed through freedom of association and expression – an agent of peace, tolerance and co-existence. It is, then, reasonable to admit that these are the fundamentals at the root of any meaningful and diversified interrelationship in any healthcare community, especially in hospitals where people from great diversity of culture, race, language, color come together to form a healing community – be it patients, physicians, nurses, social workers, dieticians, nutritionists, chaplains or spiritual / pastoral care providers, patient care technicians, transporters, radiologists, phlebotomists, and so on.

It is crucial to state that an interfaith or multi-faiths diversity in any hospital community is not, as stated above, tantamount to syncretism. That is, it is not a substitute for my faith tradition, and it is not a religion in itself. For example, when my Muslim friend visits me on Christmas and shares a meal with me and my family that does not make her/him become a Catholic Christian just as it does not convert me to the Islamic faith tradition when I visit him/her during Eid el Fitri and share in their celebration. Also, it is reasonable to believe that many hospital communities, especially high occupancy hospitals, would most definitely attract more religious representations – Judaism, Islam, Buddhist, Hindu, Christian, Baha'i, Sikh, Shinto, Zoroastrian, Jain, Confucian, Daoism, Native American, Materialism, and so on. Undoubtedly, many members of hospital communities – patients and staff – spend a great deal of time in their respective hospital community so much so that they are limited to practicing their religious beliefs there. Many observe the holy seasons of their religious traditions, for instance, the holy fasting season of Ramadan and Eid al Fitr (Islam), the holy seasons of Christmas, Lent and Easter (Christian), the feast of Krishna Janmashtami (Hindu), Rosh HaShanah and Yom Kippur (Judaism), Paryushana Parva (Jain), Navaratri (Hindu), Diwali (Hindu – Jain – Sikh), Guru Nanak Dev Sahib birthday (Sikh), and, Thanksgiving USA (Interfaith).

Admittedly, the hospital community isn't a place for religious display. However, since it has been established in our previous discussions elsewhere in this book that religion and religious practices contribute to human fulfillment and integral wholeness, it is then of unflinching importance to moderately incorporate such vital aspects of every human person, active or inactive, to the community that occupies such prominence in the here and now. Suffice it to say that hospital community isn't appropriate for proselytism. Howbeit, it should be made conducive for mutual respect of individual's beliefs and religious practices. Imposition, in whatever shape or form, would run contrary to the spirit that should permeate the healing community. Imposition could take the form of active or aggressive obligation placed on someone in his or her vulnerable state, for example, from a physician or nurse to a patient. This could occur when such a clinician directly or passively obligates the patient placed in his/her care to share his/her (clinician) beliefs. Moving contrary to this could result in a ruptured relationship between the care-seeker and the care provider. I received a call some years ago, while I was the on-call chaplain, from a nurse who requested a copy of the Christian Bible for her patient. I did ask the nurse if she would want me to bring it up to her nursing unit or…She quickly interjected, "I'll come down to get it." About fifteen minutes later, she knocked. As I handed her the Bible, she said, "Can I have two more? I give Bibles to all of my patients. I just believe that they should read it." And the question is: "How would an atheist-patient feel when s/he is presented with the Bible?" How about a disgruntled Christian! Within that same period, I worked with an intern-chaplain – a Clinical Pastoral Education student. She apparently was a devout Catholic. A report came about this zealous chaplain who was invited to the NICU (Neonatal Intensive Care Unit), one of the clinical units assigned to her. A Baptist mom, sitting by the bedside of her baby, asked the chaplain-intern to pray with her. They both held hands as she (the chaplain) recited the Rosary while the mom repeated after her.

That was a case of aggressive imposition – subtle proselytization. There could also be another form of imposition of one's "faith" or religious disposition / ideology on the vulnerable patients or subordinate hospital workers. This is in the form of denying the patient, for instance, his/her requests for religious services and supports. Sometimes, the facial expression from the attending doctor or the assigned nurse gives them away. In the course of my routine visits to a patient, it was spiritually distressing that the patient had requested the service of a chaplain for the past three days since her hospitalization but to no avail. Several excuses can be made for this systemic failure, but the bottom line remains that the patient's noble requests fell on deaf ears. It is not unusual to encounter clinicians who might not share a patient's religious worldview. Some might even consider it ridiculous when a critically ill patient recourses to spiritual support. Such clinicians' dispositions to spiritual issues or requests emanate from their *religio-psycho* worldview. However, it is a worldview that ought to be private and respect religious boundaries between the client (patient) and the care provider.

Interestingly, similar concerns are being discussed in medical forum. As published by the Advisory Board Company (June 11, 2012) "'Doctor, will you pray with me?'" in which "The University of Chicago Program on Medicine and Religion's conference in May [2012] addressed the issue of whether or not doctors should pray with their patients."[46] According to the *Journal of General Internal Medicine*, a survey (2003) that sought to measure patient preferences around prayer during their care revealed that two-thirds of respondents felt that their doctor should know about their spiritual beliefs, half said they would wish to pray with a physician in a near-death situation, and about 20% of patients liked the idea of praying during a routine office visit. From physicians' standpoint, however, a 2006 survey of 1,200 physicians in *Medical Care* found that physicians can be leery of joining patients in prayer. Fifty-three percent did so only at a patient's request, while another 17% of physicians said they never pray with patients. About 43% of responding physicians said they had no religious affiliations or are not very religious.[47] Albeit, American Medical News reports: "only 6% of physicians believe that spirituality can prevent negative outcomes among patients, although research indicates that religious individuals can have superior health outcomes."[48] This is an appropriate discourse in an appropriate arena! When I posed the same question – "Doctor, will you pray with me?" – to one of the physicians in the hospital where I work, she said, "That feels awkward!" The awkwardness of the request might be the individual's fear of "being converted" to another religious belief. However, the reality is contrary. A request to "pray with me" is not tantamount to religious conversion. It may even cement the bond between the patient and the physician. It may predispose the patient to a more trusting relationship. It may be likened to when a friend of another faith invites us to their religious function. Sharing the moment does not change, essentially, what and who we are, including our beliefs. Such experiential encounter between care-seekers and care providers, as a matter of fact, challenges our recognition and acceptance and tolerance for other faiths. It stretches the clinician or the care provider beyond or out of their religious comfort zone.

Regardless of the religious conviction we hold, there are objectively-minded themes that could promote healthy conversation between clinicians and patients, among care providers (as a team) and among a diverse group of spiritual care providers (chaplains). A Few of these would include: Fear, Anxiety, Worry, Uncertainty, Love, Charity, Hospitality, Trust, Peace, Healing, Service, Kindness, Self-giving, Care-giving, Storm, Hope, Patience, Resilience, Guilt, Light amidst darkness, Unity, Suffering and Pain: Meaning, Mortality, human frailty, sickness, illness, disease, "timely" and "untimely" Death and Transition (Gift of – Life beyond mortality), Forgiveness, Reconciliation and many more.

Chapter Five

Cultural Sensitivity & Holistic Healing

"Ask not what disease the person has, But rather what person the disease has."
– William Osler

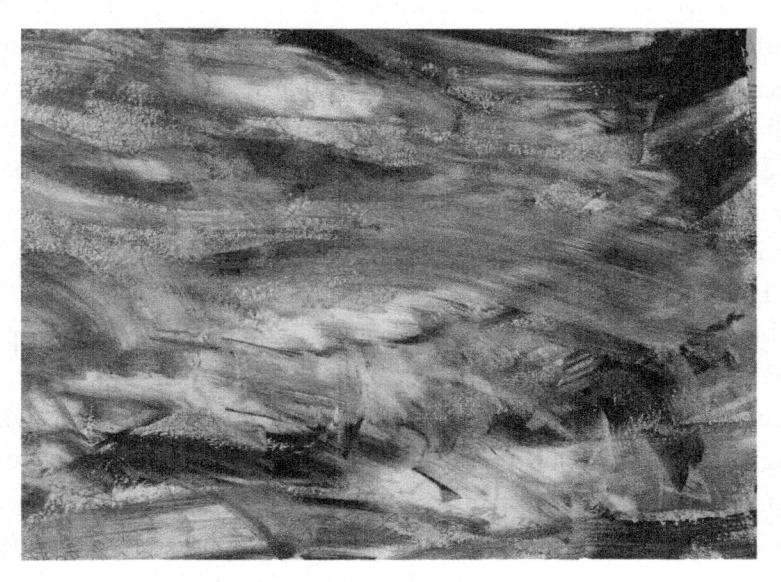

Painting by Sr. Daria Moon, SPC

It is reasonable to agree with researchers and vast number of experts who have asserted that cultural insensitivity is, most often than not, unintentional. In varied attempts to gain logical explanations for cultural insensitivity, some allusions have been made to lack of knowledge the individual or group of individuals really need in order to fully understand the other person's worldview or frame of reference. In fact, Johnson asserts: knowledge lessens anxiety, builds tolerance, honors compassion and truth. He also characterized such insensitivity as human reality about difference, about fear, about outsiders, about tribes, about others, and about powers Reminiscing, Johnson reminded his readers of the generations past, how our parents dealt with differences – different people, different nationalities, different religions, different traditions, different colors, different cultures, different foods, and different customs and practices![49]

Against the undeniable prevalence of cultural insensitivity among health care providers, in many health care settings and facilities, the policy of cultural competence remains a requirement by the Joint Commission that oversees the operational activities of hospitals and health care facilities. The Joint Commission holds hospitals accountable for addressing and maintaining patients' rights. These rights include the accommodation of cultural, religious, spiritual, and personal values as well as to religious and other spiritual practices. Consequently, The Joint Commission developed accreditation requirements for hospitals to advance effective communication, cultural competence, and patient-centered care. The implementation of this required cultural competence policy began in January 2011.

The universal creed holds that, the wholeness of the human person resides in the interconnectedness of the body, mind and spirit. They are dimensions that are integrally intertwined and inseparable without causing harm to the healthiness of the human person. Cultural values are inseparably integral to the wholeness of each human person, in sickness and in health. However, since no one can give what he or she does not have, it is reasonable to concur with Sue Wintz and Earl Cooper that in order to provide sensitive and effective holistic care, with greater respect for cultures different from the care provider's, two things have to happen: first, the care provider must be aware of his or her own cultural values, customs, and beliefs and how these influence his or her attitudes and behaviors; and second, the care provider must gain an understanding of the cultural beliefs, customs, and values of the care recipients and how they are influenced by such. Validating another person's cultural values begins with reflecting on one's own socio-cultural values, since the popular Latin maxim says: *Nemo dat quod non habet*. That is, no one gives what he or she doesn't have!

The importance of understanding and appreciating cultural

diversity in health care setting, or in any public services, cannot be overemphasized. Some authors have placed such a necessity within the context of globalization and multicultural world. For Barrett, such knowledge and appreciation of cultural diversity is called cross-cultural literacy. In fact, for Robert Rosen (2000), culturally literate leaders are apt to building cultural bridges. Cultural literacy, therefore, is the ability to understand or the knowledge gained about the fundamental differences among existing varied cultures in the world.[50]

Common Myths about Culture

- **"We are really all the same."** This is a dangerous assumption! We are certainly NOT all the same. To ensure cultural sensitivity, it is essential to acknowledge, accept, and value the differences and avoid "ethnocentrism," the tendency to believe that our own race or ethnic group is somehow better or more important than any other.

- **"I have to adopt the practices of the other culture in order to succeed."** It may be good enough to "adapt to" instead of attempting to "adopt" the practices of another culture. Adopting can result in our being misunderstood, as if mocking the culture, and thus considered disrespectful. Our decision to adopt practices of other cultures should be based on an in-depth understanding and a "thorough engagement with the culture."

- **"It's really all about personality."** While personality profiles are useful in helping us understand behavioral differences, however, drawing a direct correlation between a personality type and a culture can result in stereotypes that limit our understanding of cultural differences. Assuming that personality is the source of unfamiliar behaviors across cultures may cause a misreading of a cultural difference.

- **"I just need to be myself in order to really connect."** While we never want to violate our own sense of identity, we do need, however, to make every effort to dress and communicate both verbally and nonverbally as is appropriate to the day-to-day customs. Hence, being *"myself"* is one thing, but presenting as inappropriate and culturally insensitive within another's culture is abysmal.

Source: Walker, D., Walker, T., and Schmitz, J. (2003). *Doing Business Internationally: A Guide to Cross-Cultural Success.* New York: McGraw-Hill.

Culture & Cultural Sensitivity Defined

Culture, as a concept, has varied and numerous definitions, especially when considered from technical standpoints. Similar view holds for cultural competence as a phenomenon that portends multiple understandings and definitions especially in health care literature. When used "loosely," some consider 'culture' from geographical viewpoint, while some associate the concept with societal norms. Spencer-Oatey defined culture as "a fuzzy set of attitudes, beliefs, behavioral conventions, and basic assumptions and values that are shared by a group of people, and that influence each member's behavior and his/her interpretations of the 'meaning' of other people's behavior."[51] It is crucial to draw our attention to the key concepts used in the definition: "meaning" and "interpretations."

In an Orange Paper prepared by Lehman et al for *Mather LifeWays*, the conceptual understanding of culture was presented in a similar version as "the learned patterns of behavior and range of beliefs attributed to a specific group that are passed on through generations. It include wasy of life, norms and values, social institutions, and a shared construction of the physical world."[52] Further literature review lend credence to the previous definitions and conceptual views. In its simple form of definition, for example, culture was described as the dynamic and multidimensional context that embodies the different aspects of an individual's life. This multidimensional context includes gender, sexual orientation, profession, religion, socioeconomic status, race, and so on.[53] In all, and concurring with Barrett, culture can then be seen as the lens through which each person sees others, understands their behaviors or actions, and interpretes other people's words.

Cultural sensitivity, therefore, is defined as "the knowledge and interpersonal skills that allow providers to understand, appreciate, and work with individuals from cultures other than their own. It involves an awareness and acceptance of cultural differences, self awareness, knowledge of a patient's culture, and adaptation of skills."[54] Cultural sensitivity, otherwise known as cultural competence, describes the ability of the health care professionals to apply appropriate knowledge and professional attitudes in response to effectively meeting the care needs of all care-seekers. In demonstrating these sets of knowledge and competence, health care professionals provide "assistive, supportive, facilitative, or enabling acts that are tailor-made to fit with individual, group, or institutional cultural values, beliefs, and lifeways in order to provide quality health care."[55]

The goal of cultural sensitivity or awareness is to enhance communication between care providers and the patient and the patient's family or the caregivers. Creating an effective communication can be improved and patient care enhanced "if health care providers can bridge the divide between the culture of medicine and the beliefs and practices that make up patients' value systems."[56] For Dr. Kessler, cultural competence transcends language barriers. Nydia Gonzalez, an associate vice chancellor for institutional diversity at Tarrant County College District, opined that: "It involves sensitivity to and respect for differences in language, religion, customs, values and traditions – all these values around health care that shape the approaches that we take to health and illness."[57] Underscoring the importance of cultural sensitivity imbued with effective communication in health care settings, the Office of Minority Health – a division of the U.S. Department of Health & Human Services – has issued 14 national standards known as Culturally and Linguistically Appropriate Services (CLAS), which mandates health care organizations, especially those that receive Federal funds, to provide translation services at no cost to patients. The guidelines also calls for respectful care services to patients' "cultural health beliefs and practices and preferred language."[58]

Lehman et al underscored the relevance and the importance of cultural sensitivity or cultural awareness in health care settings, asserting that "even such concepts as health, illness, suffering, and care mean different things to different people. Knowledge of cultural customes enables health care providers to provide better care and help avoid misunderstandings among staff, residents/patients, and families."[59] Suffice it to state that cultural sensitivity or competence engenders "six aims" for quality and holistic health care: safe, effective, patient-centered, timely, efficient, and equitable.[60] The following advanatages encapsulate the benefits accruable to culturally competent health care settings:

- Enhanced or more successful patient education
- Increase in health care-seeking behavior
- Better targeted testing and screening
- Fewer diagnostic errors
- Avoidance of drug complications
- Greater adherence to medical advice[61]
- Enhanced patient's compliance level
- Reduced anxiety level
- Effective clinical time and resource management
- Better rapport and improved clinician-patient relationship – high customer relationship/satisfaction

As contended earlier, cultural sensitivity, and its corresponding effective and competent responses from the care providers in relation to health care delivery, is "necessary because even general ideas of health, illness, suffering, and care mean different thing to different groups of older adult patients."[62] It is also crucial to remember that, receiving health care services, for some minority ethnic groups such as the African Americans, could be considered as degrading or demeaning or humiliating experience, with feelings of powerlessness. Similarly, for many Chinese who find some aspects of Western medicine, such as diagnostic tests or drawing of blood, distasteful and upsetting.[63]

Factors for Major Cultural Differences

There are major elements or variables that are prevalent across cultures and also explain the existential differences. For the purpose of this book, three essential factors that would account for major differences among multicultures, especially in any health care center, will be briefly discussed. These are: context, information flow, and language. Notably, anthropologists also use these sets of variables in making distinction about culture. This book will not attempt to treat into details each of these variables, but will brief highlight key important factors of each variable for the purpose of underscoring the need for effective and holistic care through cultural sensitivity.

Context

As a student of literature class, answering a question on the "context" that led to the utterance of a statement was as synonymous as science students' tasks to balance equations in a chemistry class. Context explains the background, the environment, or the setting internally and externally that influences individuals interaction with the outside world and determines the cognitive ability to understand the words and behaviors of others. O'Hara-Devereaux and Johansen describe context as anything that surrounds, accompanies, and gives meaning to the communication.[64] It is crucial to note that cultures around the globe are divided between the low and high cultural contexts. The low-context cultures are characterized by explicit verbal messages to savor meanings in communications, with less interpersonal relationships. Such cultures rely on facts and figures, marked for **direct** and **straight-to-the point** communication style. Examples of low-context cultures include the United States and Germany.[65] High-context cultures, on the other hand, are known for extensive interpersonal relationships, placing more importance on the nonverbal messages or cues (tone, gestures, facial expressions, etc.) over and above verbal messages to understand meanings inherent in communications. High-context cultures, also known for community-oriented and group harmony as opposed to individual or individualism, often emphasize trust, intuition, and the importance of interpersonal relationships. In brief, the high-context cultures are marked for their indirect communication styles. Examples of continents or countries with such cultures include Africa, Southeast, Asia, China, and Japan.[66]

Based on the aforementioned, one can deduce that low-context cultures tend to be more direct in their choice of communication styles, while the high-context cultures are prone to use more indirect forms. **Direct-approach** cultures epitomize independence, individuality, confidence, forthrightness, and may appear authoritative and aggressive or somehow rude.[67] In contradistinction, *indirect-approach* cultures typify harmony, community togetherness, avoidance of confrontations, and may be difficult to understand their views since they express such views using indirect forms of communication. For example the *indirect-approach* cultures will rather not say "no" outrightly, but may say so using such indirect words such as, "perhaps" or "maybe,"[68] which the direct communicator may interpret as "optional." Thus, a "closed" conversation for an indirect-approach communicator is often miscontrued as "open" or "ongoing" or "negotiable" conversation by a direct-approach communicator. It is pertinent for healthcare providers, or even care receivers, to note these *slight* but profound differences between low-context and high-context cultures, direct and indirect cultural approach in communication styles. A clear understanding of the cultural context surrounding an African or Asian or Chinese patient can enhance effective communication and cultural sensitivity in the care being provided by a caucasian nurse or physician. Also, patients from high-context (indirect) cultures may not "judge" their care providers from low-context (direct) cultures as rude or too authoritative.

Information Flow

Information flow, as it relates to cultural sensitivity, typically describes how information or messages flow within an organization, as well as how individuals approach the exchanges of such information. As it pertains to the context of this book, it is crucial for both care providers and care receivers to be mindful of the nature of information flow in the clinical environment so as to ensure deeper understanding, effective care, and greater sensitivity. For instance, the United States cultural context is known for its "businesspeople type." That is, typical professional practices epitomizing such direct cultures are known for directness or "bottom-line" syndrome (in the business arena). Thus, in health care settings, such direct cultures prefer *straight-to-the-point* approach, no rigmaroling, no beating-around-the-bush, cut to the chase, and no story-telling to make a point. Communicators (patients, business partners, etc.) from indirect-approach cultures, however, may perceive this as being insensitive and always in a hurry. Effective cultural senstivity in a health care setting, therefore, will ensure that in the event of communication between two different or "opposing" cultures, communicators should create intentional flexibility and be more mindful of each other's cultural tendencies.

Language

Condon described language as the "central influence on culture and one of the most highly chareged symbols of a culture…A language does not merely record and transmit perceptions and thoughts, it actually helps to shape both."[69] In fact, Hall contended: "Culture is language; language is culture."[70] Cultural sensitivity in a health care environment will require all care providers, especially the clinicians, to be intentionally mindful of words, syntax, medical vocabularies, medical jargons, etc. and how cultures may interfere with the effective delivery of messages to the care receiver or even to a team member of a different culture.

In sum, cultural sensitivity is not an optional competence to be left at the discretional implementation of individual health professional or care provider. On the contrary, it should be *mandatorily* addressed at the organizational level. This is imperatively so given some reasons mentioned earlier. But more importantly is the fact that an organization may be deficient in meeting the totality of its vision, mission, and goals when cultural competence of its organization is deficient. For this reason, the National Center for Cultural Competence at Georgetown University sets a laudable example. The Center requires that organizations:

- ❖ Have a defined set of values and principles and demonstrate behaviors, attitudes, policies, and structures that enable them to work effectively cross-culturally

- ❖ Have the capacity to:
  - Value diversity
  - Conduct self-assessment
  - Manage the dynamics of difference
  - Acquire and institutionalize cultural knowledge
  - Adapt to the diversity and cultural contexts of the communities each hospital serves

- ❖ Incorporate the above into all aspects of policymaking, administration, practice, and service delivery and systematically invlove consumers, key stakeholders, and communities.[71]

Practical Illustrations on Cultural Differences

Illustration 1: A Case Study – Courtesy Gesture for a Bereaved Family

An African family gathered around the bedside of their loved one to say their final goodbye as the patient was about to die. The hospital, as part of its courtesy, has a culture of providing "comfort trays" containing some fruits, snacks, and drinks to the family, as part of bereavement care and support. One of the comfort trays was delivered to the dying patient's room.

Notable Cultural Difference

In the course of providing spiritual care to the patient and her family, a family member actually requested that the fruit tray and drinks be removed from the room. **Why?** According to them (African cultures), food and drinks are associated with happy mood and there's nothing to be happy about when a loved one is dying.

Suggestion: Due to some unpleasant reactions that I have seen expressed by bereaved families, I consider it paramount not to conclude this chapter on cultural sensitivity without discussing this aspect of care, concerns, love, and courtesy that hospital units, not all, often show to mourners in the heat of their impending or actual loss, cries and wailings. For the reason of cultural differences, it is appropriate to **ask** families of the deceased or actively dying patient if it is okay to serve them fruit-tray and drinks. This is symptomatic of how different cultures understand, accept, and view death and dying. While some cultures, for instance Africa and Asia (high-context cultures), may not appreciate food and drinks while their loved one is actively dying or had just died, it may be culturally acceptable for North American or German cultures (low-context cultures).

Illustration 2: A Case Study – Pain Tolerance

A 27 year old Vietnamese woman was in active labor with very strong and closely spaced contractions. The baby was positioned a little high and there was the possibility of cesarean section. Despite her difficulties, she cooperates with the doctor's instructions and labors in silence. The only signs of pain or discomfort were her look of concentration and her white knuckles.

Notable Cultural Difference

Traditional Vietnamese women, as most traditional Asians, believe that a woman must experience pain and discomfort as part of childbirth. To express these feelings, however, brings shame upon her. It might be very upsetting for an Asian woman accustomed to controlling her pains and emotions around labor and childbirth to go through labor near a highly expressive woman, or to the dismay of her care providers who are from another cultures.[72] The illustration demonstrates how different people may react to pains and discomforts in the health care setting. This may help in the pain management of patients. The care team should include cultural influence in assessing the level of pain tolerance, or not, when caring for patients, especially those from other cultures with significant tolerance for pain.

Illustration 3: A Case Study – Good Intention, Bad Omens…

A South Asian woman who has just given birth refuses to cuddle him. In fact, she barely provided minimal care – the most important care – such as feeding and changing his diaper. A chaplain, who had stopped by at the request of a staff, somehow felt sorry for the "neglected" baby. The chaplain remarked how cute the baby was, and then reached over to place her hand on the baby's head to stroke his hair. Both parents of the baby became visibly upset.

Notable Cultural Difference

This mom's apparent neglectful behavior does not reflect poor bonding. On the contrary, the seeming "distance" actually indicates a cultural belief and tradition. Many people in rural areas of South Asia believe in spirits. They believe these spirits are attracted to infants and are likely to steal them by death. Hence, the parents do everything possible not to attract attention to their newborn. Contrary to surface perceptions by other cultures, such as the chaplain's, the apparent "lack of interest or love" actually reflects an intense love and concern for the child. Not only did the chaplain attract attention to the child, but also the chaplain touched the baby in a taboo area. ***Why?*** The head is viewed by Southeast Asians as private and personal; it is the seat of the soul and is not to be touched.[73]

Suggestion: The chaplain, in the case discussed above, could be any other care provider in any hospital or health care centers. Reaching out to touch patients, babies or adults (except for immediate care providers such as nurses or physicians or for the purpose of medical examination), is not generally acceptable in all cultures. Over-assumption can compromise good intention. Hence, the chaplain could have asked: "Is it okay to touch him?" Asking politely for such permission to "*invade*" someone's space is a demonstration of cultural and professional competence.

Useful Tips on Cultural Competence

- **Be open and respectful.** Remember the rule of thumb: no culture is better, no culture is wrong, and all cultures are valuable! Cultures, whether low or high contexts, are simply different. Variety is the spice of life, the old saying goes. So, we can say of the invaluable and rich differences about cultures in the world. Be open and think outside of the box.

- **Be familiar with others' social customs.** Ignorance is not an excuse! Be familiar with the custom tenets of other cultures, especially of the cultural demographics of the people you work or interact with. "Do as Romans do" is not only when you are physically present in *Rome*, but it also means knowing and respecting the social customs associated with *Rome* (as a physical location) and with individuals wherever you may meet them.

- **Knowledge is Power.** Knowledge liberates ignorance and informs the willpower for competent and appropriate actions. As Barett rightly puts it, it is very reasonable to learn much about the culture, history, and the language of the people. This is even more imperative for health care workers, considering the multi-cultures that constitute the demographics of the patient population and the community being served. Explore the conglomeration of other continents that seek care in your organization and empower yourself with key cultural values that can be incorporated into the good and compassionate care you provide. It may be as simple as knowing countries that are Anglophone or Francophone!

- **Avoid stereotypes.** Stereotype is anti-cultural competence! Remember that there are cultures within cultures. Faces/skins may look similar, accent may sound similar; yet, origins and cultures may be far different. Hence, do not assume that every patient or co-worker from the same part of the world share the same cultural values.

Chapter Six

HOLISTIC CARE:
Spiritual Care (The Chaplain) & Medical Care (The Clinical Team)

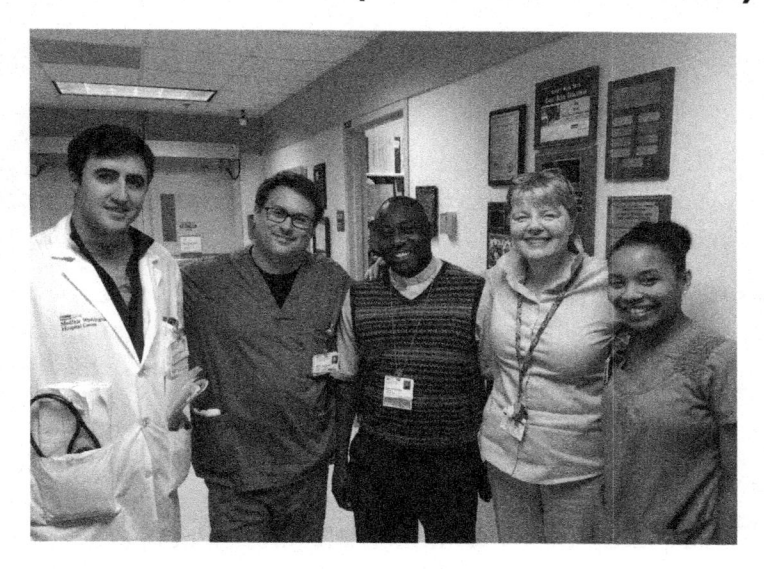

The objectives of this Chapter include:

- ❖ To understand 'Holism' as a spiritual concept
- ❖ To further understand spiritual care as a contributor to holistic healing
- ❖ To further create an awareness of spiritual care needs for patients
- ❖ To plough through the concept: "Interdisciplinary": Relevance & Goals
- ❖ To understand the possible Triggers for Spiritual Care consults

or Assessment Tool as we discern patients' spiritual care needs during clinical rounds, interdisciplinary rounds; family meetings; physician's discussion with patient, etc.

- ❖ To gain deeper understanding of the functional roles of healthcare chaplains toward a holistic goal of care.

- ❖ Finally, to enhance team spirit and collaborations with clinicians, especially as to foster prompt spiritual care consult.

Spirituality: Highlights

- ❖ A personal search for meaning and purpose in life, which may or may not be related to religion.

- ❖ It entails connection to self-chosen and/or religious beliefs, values and practices that give meaning to life, thereby inspiring and motivating individuals to achieve their optimal being.

- ❖ The results include an awareness and acceptance of hardship and mortality, a heightened sense of physical and emotional well-being, and the ability to transcend beyond the infirmities of existence.

- ❖ Giving professional attention to the subjective spiritual and religious worlds of the care receiver. Such worlds are comprised of perceptions, assumptions, feelings, and beliefs concerning the relationship of the sacred to the individual's life journey or story, situation, illness, hospitalization, recovery or possible death.

- ❖ Giving attention, care, and concern to the totality of the human person, including all that makes meaning, adds value to the person's life, and what connects the person's temporal world to the transcendental.

- ❖ Many people have remarked: "I'm not religious…but spiritual." Truly, every human person may not be religious but spiritual, having a form of connection to the Divine, the Transcendent Being.

Holistic Healing

Holism

The term 'holistic' from the Greek '*Holos*' means whole or complete. Holism is concerned with the interrelationship of body, mind and spirit in an ever-changing environment. Hutchison opines that holism is used in the present day healthcare to describe every human person as a bio-psycho-social unit. The American Holistic Nurses Association defines wellness as "that state of harmony between body, mind and spirit." The essence of holistic care is to help **"a person attain or maintain wholeness in all dimensions of their being."** In maintaining or attaining this, health providers would then need to pay attention to each of these dimensions.

Restoration

Holistic goal of care seeks to restore. Govier described the "5 Rs of spirituality": Reason, Reflection, Religion, Relationships, and Restoration. Restoration occupies a vital spot in holistic care.

- Restoration refers to the ability of a person's spirituality to have a positive influence on the physical aspects of a person.
- Alterations and changes in disposition or mood portend a need for restoration.
- Such alterations can impact the plan of care for patients or optimal service of clinicians or associates.
- In the overall holistic goal of care in any hospital, clinical staff or associates or administrators can access spiritual /pastoral care department for supportive restoration of spiritual wellbeing.

Certain life events can cause an inability to "restore" the body to a spiritual equilibrium, resulting in spiritual distress. A patient or an associate may manifest some changes in disposition or mood, emotions or physical being. Whatever the alteration, the clinical staff should be able to recognize signs of spiritual distress and draw on either personal or adjunctive means to assist the patient or associate in restoring spiritual wellbeing.[74]

Clinicians' Views on Spiritual Care for Patients[75]

A total of 4,000 nurses were surveyed (April, 2010) and the following statements reveal some intriguing views expressed to underscore the need of spiritual care for their patients:

- "I consider spirituality to be part of the 'whole' care one should be giving to patients and families. To me it means ensuring that the 'mind', i.e. thoughts, worries etc, as well as the body, is considered when providing care."

- "It would be very hard to find a nurse who saw only the physical aspect of care as that which defines nursing. We all know that when a person is hurting emotionally, all sorts of physical ailments crop up. On the other hand, physical conditions can affect the mind and spirit."[76] (Hutchison, 1997).

In addition to these laudable views, the surveyed nurses also described what 'spiritual care' would mean for them and for their patients:

- 94% favor respect for privacy, dignity and religious and cultural beliefs.
- 90% feel that providing spiritual care improves the overall quality of nursing care.
- 83% believe spirituality is a fundamental aspect of nursing, even for patients with no religious beliefs.
- 80% feel that the need for spiritual care also applies to atheists and agnostics.
- 91% of nurses believe that they can provide spiritual care

- 94% do not believe that spirituality involves only going to church or a place of worship.[77]

Historical Background of Healthcare Chaplaincy[78]

Biblical Foundation

In the Hebrew Scripture, aka Old Testament, the Book of Joshua, Levite priests accompany the Israelites' military and political expedition into Israel, carrying the Ark of the Covenant and playing a major role in the goodwill of military matters. While these priests cannot be considered "chaplains" with the current meaning, their role as spiritual aides provides a model for modern chaplains to rely upon.[79] The religious practice of involving the priest, for intercessory roles and spiritual aides, continued throughout the history of the early Christian community. A profound indication and instruction was given by Apostle James: "Is anyone among you suffering? He should pray. Is anyone in good spirits? He should sing praise. Is anyone among you sick? He should summon the presbyters of the church, and they should pray over him and anoint [him] with oil in the name of the Lord, and the prayer of faith will save the sick person, and the Lord will raise him up. If he has committed sins, he will be forgiven" (Jm 5: 13-15).

Not only this but the care for the sick, the afflicted, the needy and the poor occupied the central public ministry of Jesus Christ, as recorded in Matt 8, 9; Mk 3: 1-6, 5, 6: 53-56, 7: 31-37; Lk 4: 38-41, 14: 1-6; Jn 9, 11, etc, examples of which the church and His ardent disciples are encouraged to follow. These biblical injunctions have always formed the foundation of integrating the care for the sick into the pastoral responsibilities of the "presbyters" (college of priests). Thus, such care allows the elders of the faith-community to reach out to the ailing members of their flock for which they were solely responsible.

The term chaplain comes from the fourth century legend, Martin of Tours.[80] Martin was born to a pagan family about 316 A.D. in Pannonia, a Roman province that included modern Hungary. When he grew up, he became a Roman soldier. At approximately age 21, on a very cold winter day, Martin was passing by the gates of Amiens in Gaul (what is today France). He saw a man who was freezing by the side of the road. He was moved with compassion after seeing and hearing the pleas of the beggar being ignored by several others who had ridden by on their horses. He decided to help, though he had little himself. He took the one valuable possession he owned — his cape — and cut it in half with his sword. He kept half for himself and gave the other half to the beggar. That night, as the story goes, Martin had a vision in which he came to understand that the beggar was Christ Himself. The vision shook Martin to the core. After that experience, he decided to follow the Christian faith and was baptized by Bishop St. Hillary. Ultimately, he left the army to devote himself to the church. He later became Bishop of Tours and founded a monastery in Eastern Europe. After his death, the remaining half of the cape became a relic — an object of value as a religious reminder of his life and work. The cloak (Latin: *cappa*) was kept in a shrine and eventually the place took on the name of the cape. The French took the word into their language as *chapele,* from which comes the English word chapel. During the Middle Ages, St. Martin's cloak was carried into battle by the kings as a banner signifying the presence of God. But since it was a sacred relic of the church, a priest went along as custodian. This guardian of the cape, or *capellanus* (which became chaplain in Old French) also tended to the king's religious needs. This is where the word chaplain comes from. It gives a clue into the essential nature of the chaplaincy, explaining the origin of the terms "chaplain" and "chapel" as we know it today.[81]

Historically, the chaplain was a member of one institution — the church — serving another institution, the army. Definitions of the chaplaincy seldom take into account this institutional duality. However, the history of chaplaincy development has continually evolved so much so that many other religious institutions, such as Jewish Faith Tradition, provide such noble spiritual and pastoral services for their believers. While some other religious affiliates encourage their interested members, through endorsements, to acquire the professional skills of providing spiritual support to the sick – Clinical Pastoral Education (CPE). Howbeit, suffice it to say that chaplains in the healthcare field are unique in that they are the only member of the medical team whose primary identification is with a non-medical institution. They are also unique in their religious institutions as the only ministers who are professionally certified and endorsed to serve in a healthcare institution.[82] It is essential to mention that there are different kinds of chaplains:

- ❖ **Domestic Chaplains:** A domestic chaplain was a chaplain attached to a noble household in order to grant the family a degree of self-sufficiency in religion. The chaplain was freed from any obligation to reside in a particular place so he could travel with the family, internationally if necessary, and minister to their spiritual needs. Domestic chaplains performed family christenings, funerals and weddings and were able to conduct services in the family's private chapel, excusing the nobility from attending public worship.[83]

- ❖ **Military Chaplains:** The first English military-oriented chaplains were priests on board proto-naval vessels during the eighth century A.D. Land-based chaplains appeared during the reign of King Edward I, although their duties included jobs that today would come under the jurisdiction of military engineers and medical officers. A priest attached to a feudal noble household would follow his liege lord into battle. In 1796 the Parliament of Great Britain passed a Royal Warrant that established the Royal Army Chaplains' Department in the British Army. The current form of military chaplain dates from the era of World War I. A chaplain provides spiritual and pastoral support for service personnel, including the conduct of religious services at sea or in the field. In the Royal Navy, chaplains are traditionally addressed by their Christian name, or with one of many nick-names (Bish; Sin-Bosun; Devil Dodger; Sky-Pilot; God Botherer etc). In the British Army and Royal Air Force, chaplains are traditionally referred to (and addressed) *as padre*. In 1865, Abraham Lincoln signed legislation establishing the first national Homes for Disabled Volunteer Services. Chaplains were paid a salary of "$1500 per year and forage for one horse."

The Veterans Administration established chaplaincy services for all of their hospitals in 1945.

- **Corporate Chaplains:** Some businesses, large and small, employ chaplains for their staff and/or clientele. According to *The Economist* (August 25, 2007, p. 64) there are 4,000 corporate chaplains in the US alone, with the majority being employees of specialist chaplaincy companies such as Marketplace Chaplains, USA. According to the company, turnover at Taco Bell outlets in central Texas dropped by a third after they started employing chaplains. Another organization supplying chaplains to corporations is Corporate Chaplains of America. CCA was founded in 1996 to provide genuine "Caring in the Workplace," while following a structured business plan built upon process management principles. The organization employs full time, long term, career chaplains who combine workplace experience with professional chaplaincy training.

- **Various Chaplains:** Chaplains also can be attached to sports teams, emergency service agencies, educational institutions, police and fire departments, private clubs, scout troops, ships, prisons, and nightclubs. The term can also refer to priests attached to Roman Catholic convents.

- **Healthcare Chaplains:** In a healthcare facility, a chaplain ministers primarily to the spiritual needs of patients/residents, family members, staff, and as an encourager to local pastors. The chaplain may serve as a volunteer or s/he may be an employee of the healthcare facility.[84]

Over the years of its evolution, hospital chaplaincy has gained greater prominence as studies have substantiated the fundamental truth about every human as bio-psycho-social beings. The advancement of Western medicine has occurred, not just in technological equipments, but also in the understanding and integration of the spiritual dimension of the human person to the care being provided at healthcare facilities. Also, healthcare is better served through the enriched services of other supportive disciplines. It is commonsensical that most patients, if not all, from the moment of admission till discharge (either to their respective homes or facility centres) are in need of a combination of professional services: physician, nurse, social worker (case manager), chaplain, dietician, ethicist, and PT/OT (Physiotherapist/Occupational Therapist). Some might need additional specialities such as psychiatrist, language interpreter, etc. This representation of multi-disciplines, otherwise called interdisciplinary team, work to achieve a common goal: a holistic healing of every patient that passes through the healthcare facility. It is amazing, nonetheless, to witness the interaction among these clinical and non-clinical multi-disciplines. Such an interface corroborates the claim that medicine and healing employs a combination of approaches according to the multidimensional aspects of the creature: human being.

Holistic Care as a mission for the Interdisciplinary Care Team[85]

The focus of any interdisciplinary team in any health care setting is to provide and enhance holistic care for the patients. This is the singular goal of the multi-professional eyes looking out for one common outcome. Interdisciplinary is "the ability to analyze, synthesize and harmonize links between disciplines into a coordinated and coherent whole," as defined by the Canadian Institutes of Health Research (CIHR, 2005). Similarly, the University of New Hampshire states that interdisciplinary "integrates the knowledge and perspectives of multiple areas of expertise to holistically solve problems..." (2004). It can be deduced, from these two substantive definitions, that interdisciplinary underscores the integration of concepts "from different disciplines" geared toward achieving a synthesis of a "co-ordinated coherent whole." For the purpose of this volume, and its practical application in healthcare industry, especially in hospital settings, 'interdisciplinary' would be defined as a coalesced team efforts among several professional care providers that seek to collaborate and contribute informed knowledge for the purpose of attainable holistic care and healing of patients in their care.

It is pertinent to state that the relevance and invaluable nature of an interdisciplinary team has been widely embraced by most hospitals, if not all, and other health care facilities. It is further underscored by some institutes of learning, such as Northern Arizona University, in establishing the 'Interdisciplinary Health Policy Institute.' Its Founding Principle is worth quoting in this article: "The Interdisciplinary Health Policy Institute is founded on the principle that strategic partnerships and interdisciplinary teams most effectively meet today's health and health care challenges." In my years of experience in hospital ministry, the need for an interdisciplinary care team has slowly but progressively been embraced by hospitals, contextualizing such need to each hospital structure and operative strategy. The driving force, evidently, is to arrive at a well-coordinated common goal of care for the good of the patient. This driving force is clearly palpable among the five different hospitals in which I have ministered on the East coast of North America.

At the heart of this interdisciplinary formation resides the striking realization of the multi-facets or dimensions of a human person. It is unarguably true that every human person is physical or biological; psycho-social (emotions, moral sense, intellect and will); and, spiritual (transcending physical and psychosocial dimensions). These are considered as the three overlapping dimensions of a human person. Hence, a hospitalized person would thus have many needs according to different segments or dimensions of her or his life. It might, then, become a disservice to focus on only one dimension – say, the physical. It is not unthinkable that the physical state, which mostly brings people to a health care facility, might sometimes be contingent on the level of attention given to other essential areas affecting the care seeker. By this it means, the physical healing might be accelerated or decelerated depending on the level of attention given to the *"total"* person, say, the contributory roles of nutritionist, physical therapist, chaplain, social worker, ethicist, etc. Rather than segregated or disintegrated care plans, a care-seeker would benefit more from a complete and holistic care "package." Think of a patient who refused further care unless his physical hunger (food) was attended. The attending physician and other clinicians felt frustrated as the patient's "uncooperative" attitude stalled further action. It took the listening presence of a chaplain to "figure out" the immediate need of the patient: "I'm weak! No food, no further procedure…" voiced the patient and family. It might sound quite simplistic, but the scenario demonstrates team collaboration premised on one vision, one mission and one goal. Around the interdisciplinary table is a team comprised of: Attending physician; nurse; case manager; social worker; spiritual/pastoral care; bioethics specialist; nutrition; PT/OT etc, deliberate on care plan for each patient per the nursing unit concerned. Sharing their informed knowledge about the patient, each discipline uses its skilled measures to evaluate the patient. Such an approach affords team members good understanding of the patient's relevant past medical history, the present situation and/or condition, plan/goal of care while hospitalized, as well as a discharge plan. Every discipline contributes a little to result in a "mighty healing."

As a chaplain, one might ask, how do I contribute to the interdisciplinary care plan to herald holistic healing for patients? In the collaborative effort with other clinical disciplines, the attentiveness of a chaplain would help in identifying some important triggers for spiritual care involvement. This can be referred to as 'the triggers for spiritual/pastoral care consult' or simply, the assessment tool. The following can provide necessary and better understanding for clinicians to know when to consult spiritual/pastoral care department, as well as what chaplains listen for during their participation in interdisciplinary rounds. It is pertinent to state that these fourteen triggers are assessment tools that can enhance chaplains' contribution to the holistic goal of care for patients and/or family members. The tools can as well facilitate seamless professional collaboration between clinicians and chaplains. However, it is crucial to state that the list is not exhaustive.

Triggers for a Spiritual Care Consult: An Assessment Tool for Clinicians[86]

Spirituality Expressed in Religions

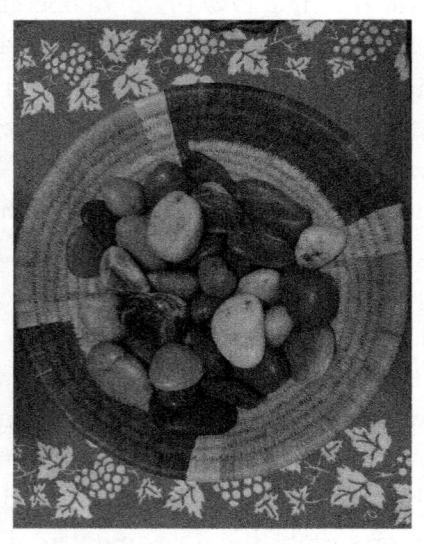

Patients, families and clinicians may express their spirituality through their religions and religious affiliations. In most hospitals or facilities where spiritual care services are provided, it is imperative to welcome, respect and provide support for all faith traditions. The religious symbols shown above represent major faith traditions commonly found in the demographics of patients as well as the dynamics of the workforce. As the hospital community is enriched with a vast diversity of culture and race, so also will its enrichment extend to multi-religious and non-religious affiliates. Suffice it to say that institutions of care providers, like any other public institution of establishment, are obliged to respect the freedom of religious association and expression of faith.

Trigger #1: Change in Code Status

- AND/DNR (Allow Natural Death / Do Not Resuscitate)
- Comfort Care
- ⬥ Palliative Care
- ⬥ Hospice (home or facility)

When the goal of care changes from aggressive / curative care to comfort care, conversations necessarily have to change in the new direction of care. Patients and family members would need some emotional and spiritual support as they deal with acceptance and the new reality. Spiritual Care should be contacted whenever a patient's goal of care changes either by medical order or at the patient's or family's decision. The chaplain can assist patient or family members to process the new direction in their goal of care and importantly, to gradually initiate an end-of-life conversation with the patient or caregivers. Comfort measure, undoubtedly, may present a distressing situation as much as receiving sad news. Reactions and feelings may vary in response to this direction of care. For patients and families who feel extremely devastated, especially at the physician's order, could benefit from the spiritual support offered by the chaplain. Some hospitals, as a matter of fact, operate on a policy that would necessitate that the nursing unit informs spiritual care department in the event that the patient's code status has changed from aggressive care to comfort care. This timely and appropriate interdisciplinary continuous care will be helpful to all, especially the patient and family members.

Trigger #2: **Complete or partial shut-down**

- Patient shuts down
- Patient is less communicative or engaging

Patient's disposition can change for a number of reasons. The change in mood and disposition might be related to the patient's hospitalization and it might not. Whatever the reason and cause might be, when a patient shuts down or becomes less engaging or communicative, it can be an indication that something is happening in his/her inner world. It is a physical manifestation of the inner trouble or conflict, yearning for resolution and help. I was once consulted for an oncology patient who was said to be "depressed" because of his cancer diagnosis and subsequent chemotherapy treatment plan. On stopping by, I engaged the patient in a spiritual care chat. Mr. Giugno was sad and troubled, neither for the reason of his diagnosed health situation nor regarding the "scary" treatment plan. Rather, he was deeply troubled because he was engaged in a conflict with his girlfriend prior to his hospital visit. The conflict led to putting her out of the house. Then he locked the house and came to the hospital with the house key. He had thought, as he said, that his hospital visit was going to be 'in-and-out'. Unfortunately, he had been kept in hospitalization for the past five days. He said he was deeply worried about the safety of his girlfriend, wondering where she could be staying since his hospitalization. As Mr. Giugno sat at the edge of his hospital bed, he was seemingly filled with thoughts, concerns, perhaps guilt, etc. This is a typical case in which a patient could be troubled, distressed or saddled with life situations that are not, strictly speaking, related to the immediate health issues but some other concerns – social or family related. Situations, like Mr. Giugno's or the likes, could be assuaged as a result of the chaplain's listening ear to help figure out what is ruling the patient's world here and now. It is pertinent to say that patients or families are more disposed to discussing such or similar issues with chaplains than with physician or nurse. Working with the patient can possibly turn a moody situation into a cheerful one, from partial or complete shut-down to a more engaging or communicative care-receiver as Mr. Giugno eventually turned out to be. Spiritual Care, as a resource, will be of great help to get the patient back on track.

Trigger #3: **Denial or Reluctance to accept the reality of**

Health condition or deteriorating terminal health condition
- ◇ Coping mechanism
- ◇ Unrealistic expectation
- ◇ Miracle "syndrome"

Denial or acceptance of health condition or health prognosis can be difficult, both for patients and/or families. It can be symptomatic of a broken heart. Hence, there is the tendency not to accept or deny the reality, especially when it is "sudden." Some patients or family members could employ this as a coping mechanism, intentionally or not. Sometimes, it may portray an unrealistic goal or expectation that the patient or family members place on the physician or care team. Also, patient or families may tap into faith or spirituality to find possible answers to the present disturbing reality. Such answers may include the expectation of a miracle against all odds or medical facts. This can be difficult for clinicians and care providers. For alert and oriented patients, key expressions may include: "I'm not ready!" "I know…God will do it!" This may include unfinished "business", love for life, house not yet in order, miracle syndrome, etc. Whenever you hear any of these or similar expressions, call on a chaplain.

    I was consulted for a 62-year-old patient who was actively dying of lung disease. He was admitted to the Intensive Care Unit (ICU), hooked to a life-support ventilator, unable to sustain good blood pressure, facing multiple organ failure, etc. The patient was intubated and unconscious. His inability to actively participate in his care, especially in moments of decision-making, conferred the right on his wife. All medical updates, consents and progress reports were presented to the wife. As days went by, it became medically appropriate to change the code status of Mr. Strong to DNR/AND (Do Not Resuscitate/Allow Natural Death). His POA (Power of Attorney), the wife, reluctantly agreed. All along, Mr. Strong's wife continually maintained that her husband was not dying. Several biblical quotations in favor of resurrection and God's power to heal were often recited as she prayed devotedly over her dying husband. On one occasion, during one of my stop-bys, she anointed him with oil purposed to herald resurrection, she said. She repeatedly maintained that her husband was not dying, regardless of medical facts. To make a long story short, Mr. Strong died on the respirator. The entire clinical team, Mrs. Strong (patient's wife) and I were present as he journeyed from our corporeal world to the world beyond. The physician pronounced him dead and turned the respirator off. The monitor was also turned off. Shortly after their clinical protocol, she asked everyone to leave the room, saying: "I need to resurrect him…he's not dead." We all stepped out while prayers for resurrection continued.

    Prayer for a miracle is not unfamiliar in a hospital setting – critical or less critical situations. Such prayers can be an exercise of faith and hope. Such prayers, on the other hand, can further support the unrealistic tendency of the patient or family members, thereby deprived of the necessary preparation needed for what is about to happen. Do miracles happen in hospitals? Absolutely, yes! Do they happen all the time and in all cases? Absolutely not! On whose case is it going to happen next? Only God Almighty knows! Why does God not perform miracles all the time and in all human cases of illness or sickness? No one has an answer to that! These are fundamental theological puzzles that often ravage the human mortal world for which the chaplain can help the miracle-expectant to process. This should not give rise to ill-feeling, or disappointment or become irritated. Rather, it will be helpful if physicians or nurses or other caring clinical staff members understand that families in this type of situation are paddling a troubled boat, tossed by heavy winds amidst scary "lightning and thunderstorms" while they hope that divine intervention could reverse the rage of storms. Whatever the reasons for 'miracle-expectation' might be – cultural, faith, or spirituality – such an expectant (patient or family members) can benefit from the services of chaplains, trained to provide skillful responsive listening. Both the chaplain and patient and/or family members, then, engage and ponder on the theme "miracle" and why the miracle isn't happening as the patient or family members might expect.

Trigger #4: *"Eager"* for earthly departure

- Patient feels overwhelmed by:
    - Frequent or repeated visits to hospital
    - Unresolved medical issues
    - Age-related medical condition(s)
    - Insufficient support and Increased dependence
    - Patient feels 'enough is enough!'

It is not unusual to find this more common among geriatric patients. This can occur when a patient blatantly refuse to cooperate with a medical plan of care. However, it may seem that the patient is eager or "wish" for death. As a matter of fact, some older patients might say "I want to die." Or, it can be couched in a key expression: "I want to go home." It is important to know that "home" might possess deeper meaning than the surface interpretation that depicts a physical location. This may be due to repeated medical crises, repeated hospital visits for unresolved medical issues, etc. This is an opposite of the last trigger – 'denial or reluctance to accept...' This is typically a case in which the physicians and the medical care team truly believe that they have yet to exhaust all possible and reasonable options available to the patient but to which the patient seems not prepared to explore any further. Granted that patient's previous hospital visits did not conclude or offer conclusive diagnosis. But it may be a confirmation of the limitations of science, technology and human wisdom. When patients or loved ones feel low-spirited or discouraged by the length of time it has taken to arrive at a decisive reason for illness and subsequent plans of care, it may be a time to request a chaplain's visit. Such patients and/or family members need encouragements, words of hope, and a bridge to cross from gloominess to brightness, and from disheartened tunnel to high-spirited way forward.

Trigger #5: **Family Meeting**

- ◈ Medical updates
- ◈ Decision-oriented
- ◈ Family dynamics

A family meeting can be a good avenue by which to tap into diverse resources available to patients, families, and clinical team. Such meetings provide support both for patients and family members, as well as for the care team. Team work can better serve the needs of patients or families during family meetings for the purpose of medical updates, decision-making, and family issues that might impact care of the patient. Sometimes, a chaplain can help 'step down' loads of distressing information heaped on a patient and/or caregivers. At such meetings, especially at decision-oriented

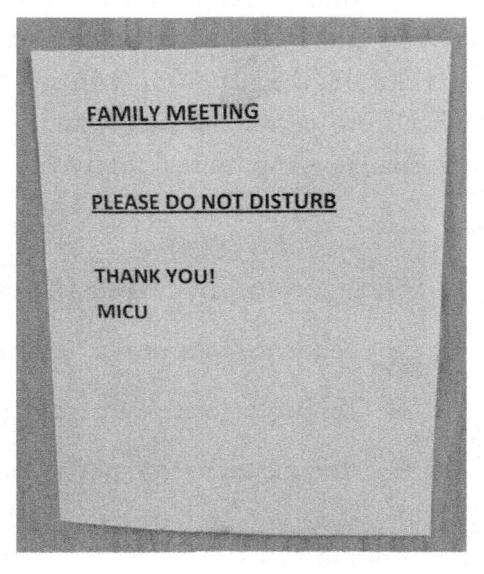

FAMILY MEETING

PLEASE DO NOT DISTURB

THANK YOU!
MICU

meetings, a chaplain's presence can further assist families to focus on other necessary aspects of the human person other than the prevailing ailment. Such "odd" conversations may include 'dying with dignity,' 'what are the patient's likes?' 'How can we, as family members, spend the remaining days qualitatively with him or her other than focusing on what more the physician can do to reverse the irreversible situation?'

Helping loved ones name some important things that their dying relative would appreciate has, most often, been a great source for strength and closure. As perceived, it may be an appropriate time to deal with forgiveness and reconciliation in the family. Or, the family meeting may help reveal that the son or daughter is struggling with a "guilt factor," either genuinely or self-imposed. For that reason, the clinical team may experience stonewalls. The calming presence of a chaplain at such meetings can be comforting. It can also help to resolve tensions between care-providers and caregivers. Brownstone captures the essence of the chaplain's presence to the patient or family when she surmised: "The pastor [or chaplain] may succeed, at times, in helping facilitate the intense emotions, express the deep thoughts, and disclose the unresolved matters and, by doing so, helping family members reach some resolution and closure. The pastor [or chaplain] may witness healing of past wounds, relief from current tensions, and emergence of fresh communication, transparency, and mutual forgiveness."

Trigger #6: Equating Illness with "Being a Burden"

- ❖ Tendency to accept a "*quick defeat*"
- ❖ Tendency to seek an "*easy way out*"
- ❖ "Independent" life not to be relinquished

Interpreting illnesses and life circumstances depend on the patient's spiritual, emotional and psychological arsenal. View about life, self and the independence of "self" are vital factors in eventual acceptance of one's new diagnosis and the need to accept others' help when needed. For patients who value their independence on a very high scale, it is not unusual to equate illness to being a burden. Such a patient might reject procedures or surgery that will make him or her depend on families or friends or a significant other. For obvious reason, s/he doesn't want to be incapacitated or dependent. Hence, he or she might seek an *"easy way out,"* which is, a rejection of such a medical care plan. Upon attentive listening, clinicians can pick up such a vibe as key expressions may include: "I don't want to obstruct anyone's life…" Or, "I don't want to be a burden to…"

I was once consulted regarding a patient who'd refused amputation due to rapidly spreading infections. The amputation was a matter of urgency and necessity to save her and prolong her life. When I visited with the patient, she agreed that the amputation would be a good idea since the infection had done damage to her leg. However, she refused, according to her, because she did "want to be a burden to anyone." "I am going to be wheelchair-bound and become a burden to my granddaughter?" she rhetorically questioned. This is seemingly a "dangerous" path to thread. The patient might be threading a thin line between embracing "avoidable death" and the choice of *"unintentional"* euthanasia. It is a spiritual-ethical dilemma for which the chaplain can be a great resource and support to the patient.

This can be understandable for the elderly who have been very independent for most of their lives. The thought of losing such independence can be very torturing. Its possibility seems more destructive than the reason for the hospitalization. The reassuring presence of a chaplain can inject spiritual insight into the storm of the moment. Often, patients and families feel the calming Divine presence amidst their turbulence whenever they pour out their troubled minds to the chaplain. The chaplain does not pretend to have answers to their worries and innumerable questions; but, the fact that the patient or caregiver could savor the non-judgmental listening presence of a spiritual figure can be a relief psychologically and emotionally.

Trigger #7: **Non-Compliance**

- ◈ Patient seems to have given up on self
    - ◈ Prospect of care/treatment

- ◈ Refuses treatment, medications, food, less engaging, etc.
- ◈ S/he displays:
  - Loss of hope
  - Less enthusiastic about everything and anything, etc.

The responses to health condition and/or situation can take different twists. It is important to note that manners of response and reactions differ from patient to patient. It can sometimes weave into emotional, psychological and spiritual responses. It is not unusual to see the patient in a critical condition, expectedly or not, giving up on oneself and the care plan, thereby refusing medications, treatments, food; etc. This can further lead to loss of hope and enthusiastic spirit. The chaplain will be a good resource to restore hope amidst "hopelessness." The chaplain does not have "extraordinary" or magical power to overturn the decision of a patient. However, the chaplain combines different levels of authority – divine and human – and his/her professional skills to engage the patient in such manner as to improve the comfort level of the patient to "open up" to the chaplain much more than he or she might do with other care providers.

Mr. Suite was said to be non-compliant during his hospitalization at one of the hospitals in which I worked. His compliance issue was that he consistently refused his blood pressure medication. His nurse had had conversations with him several times to no avail. I was "accidentally" involved in the case while on the nursing unit for other purposes. My spiritual care conversation with Mr. Suite revealed that the medication was a "trigger" for him. He said: "That was the same medication that killed my wife two years ago…I'm not gonna take it." Caring for the well-being – mind, body and spirit – (spiritual care) of the patient, sometimes, reaches beyond the confines of the patient's bed space or the hospital as a whole. This is premised on the fact that the patient's decision to do or not to do, to be compliant or not compliant, is more often than not informed by their past memories and present life issues. Hence, spending time to listen to patients' stories, which physicians rarely have time for due to their busy schedule, helps to uncover deep reasons behind the choices they make. For the most part, "solutions" or the probable way forward is contained in the very story the patient shares. That is, listening to the patient helps the patient to listen to himself or herself. It is also a form of empowerment and validation. The chaplains can truly be your "listening ears" to foster the healing most desired by the patient.

Trigger #8: Fear & Anxiety

- The fear of the unknown destination
- Anxiety over family and management of estates
- Concern about family or an "individual"
- Anxiety and concerns over:
    - Surgery or Procedure
    - Amputation
    - Tumor/cancerous growth
    - Transplant, etc.

The fear of the unknown destination, concerns about life after death, the fear of death itself is not unusual for patients to express anxiety and concern over their families as well as the management of estates should death occurs. The hospitalization might be so sudden that it never afforded the patient any time to put her house in order. Some male patients have expressed worry over what might happen to their wives as they battle with their critical or life-threatening health situations. Some needed to hear it – reassurance – from their spouses that "I'll be fine," "Children or kids will be fine," "We'll be fine," "Things will be alright." The thought of knowing: "all will be well and fine" even if the patient dies can be very comforting and calming to patients experiencing such anxiety and worry. Many a time, patients share these worries and concerns with the chaplain and not with the spouse. Sometimes, also, mothers share their concerns, with the chaplain, over the "age-long" conflict among their children. Not only may thoughts of this nature dampen their spirits, but such legitimate concerns could also impact their healing and recovery process – blood pressure, heart rate, etc. Expressions such as "I'm not concerned about myself but…" might be indicative of worry of some sort over other family member(s) – anxiety that bothers the patient and about which he or she might be disposed to talk.

Finally, anxiety and concerns in view of impending surgery/procedure (amputation, tumor/cancerous growth, transplant, etc) can be troubling to patients or family members. Some hesitations can be attributed to the fear of surgeon's knife, or simply the fear of surgery: tomophobia. While physicians converse with their patients, it may be helpful to call on the chaplain whenever this key expression, or similar expressions, ensues: "I'm afraid..!" Or, "I don't know how this will turn out." Although it should be noted that chaplains do not possess magical power to "arm-twist" patients in changing their minds. However, chaplains walk in their pastoral authority that often enables calming and resolving atmosphere for patients and even in an utterly confused situation. Empowering the patient, through an art of responsive listening, often help the patient to self-proffer "way-out" of the perceived "clumsy" situation. In brief, a chaplain's presence can be helpful in a situation like this. However, care should be taken in offering such a resource to the patient as it may also aggravate fear, panic and induce a trust issue. Clinicians should offer spiritual care service as a "support service" within the care team and not as an extraordinary agent called to *pray so that…* " The attending physician can say something like: "Ms. Tama, will it be helpful if you **discuss** this care plan (fear or concern) with a chaplain?"

The spiritual care service is a continuation of the holistic care being offered to the patient and her family. When offered as a seamless team care, there is a high probability, based on experience, that acceptance and favorable disposition are assured.

Trigger #9: **Mere coincidence but impactful memory**

- ◈ Same hospital
- ◈ Same patient care unit
- ◈ Same room
- ◈ Similar medical diagnoses

- ◆ Similar illness and health condition
- ◆ Same age
  - As deceased relative – son, daughter, mom, dad, sister, brother, etc.

We understand that life is full of coincidences. However, some coincidences can impact patients' care and holistic healing. It is not uncommon to have a patient whose family members or relations have once been hospitalized at the same hospital or healthcare facility. In some peculiar situations, some might have lost dad, mom, daughter, son, granddad, grandma, granddaughter, grandson, nephews or nieces, sisters or brothers to the same diagnosis at the same hospital, same nursing unit and sometimes, even the same unit room. Such memories can have a great impact. I was consulted on a case in which a patient was dying of leukemia. The family meeting – with his dad – was set up in a free room on the nursing unit. The meeting was brief and very informative for the patient's dad. After the clinicians left, however, I sat with him for more spiritual counseling. In the course of our conversation, he shared that he had lost a daughter – patient's older sibling – to leukemia (same cancer diagnosis) two years earlier, here (same hospital), inside the same room in which we were sitting (same nursing unit, same room). For a few seconds, I was startled! He motioned and whispered words that could hardly be expressed, to indicate "this room." Tears and trembling were all I could see. What a story! Some patients have similar stories. The thought of dealing with the same diagnosis of a deceased member of their family can be a nightmare. Those feelings can hinder the peace of mind that is necessary to focus on the plan of care. The chaplain can help the patient process these "coincidence of life ordeals" thereby enabling the patient to focus on his or her health and possible recovery, if God wills.

Trigger #10: Recent loss / Series of losses

- ◆ In the family prior to or...
- ◆ During hospitalization

The stormy sea of life can sometimes become too turbulent! When a patient's story includes incidents of recent deaths or series of deaths in the family, the turbulent waves certainly need a calming and comforting presence of a spiritual care provider. The patient may spend more time dealing with the grief(s), thereby shifting focus from self-care or care plan. The patient may feel that s/he has "too much to handle" thereby facing possible risk of spiritual distress. Depending on the level of relationship between the patient and the deceased family member, the level of emotional and spiritual trauma can be significant. This can affect the patient's peace of mind thereby causing psychological restlessness and its consequent effects on blood pressure and heart rate. The bereaved needs grief counseling to deal with the loss in order to bring back the focus to the goal of care.

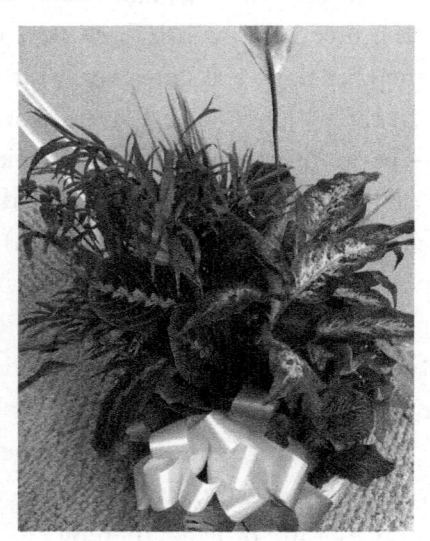

The Trigger #11: Sad medical news

- Difficult medical diagnosis
- Poor prognosis
    - Brain death,
    - Irreversible damage,
    - Multiple organ failure, etc.

It is customary that recipients of sad news – medical or in other areas of life – rely on supports from friends and families to get through their difficult moments. After all, the Bible exhorts: "Blessed are they who mourn, for they will be comforted" (Matt 5: 4). It is also true that the period of medical tests can be a "long waiting" period! Patients and/or families can be anxious about the results of their diagnostic tests. When the result seems to confirm possible fears, or might bring sadness to patients and/or families, there is a need for spiritual support from the chaplain. Also, in the event of poor prognosis after the diagnostic test, families or patients can make use of spiritual care support, as they deal with the reality of chronic or acute illness before them. To the patient or caregivers, such a sad news or poor prognosis can be viewed as a loss. If so, then, comforting them will seem appropriate. For instance, a patient suffers subarachnoid hemorrhage. A brain (cerebral) aneurysm is a bulging, weak area in the wall of an artery that supplies blood to the brain. In most cases, a brain aneurysm causes no symptoms and goes unnoticed. In rare cases, the brain aneurysm ruptures, releasing blood into the skull and causing a stroke. When a brain aneurysm ruptures, the result is called a subarachnoid hemorrhage. Depending on the severity of the hemorrhage, brain damage or death may result.[87] This is not a place anyone wants to be! Families are often distraught when their loved one is faced with the reality of severe and irreversible brain damage or the patient is declared brain dead. It can be more shocking and even traumatic when no prior symptom was noticed.

Trigger #12: **Slow response/consent (or pessimism)**

- Patient refuses to give/sign consent
- Patient "pretends" not to understand physician or care team on health issues
- Patient asks repeated questions, especially same question(s) from different care providers

Sometimes a patient or family member may experience "information overload" as a result of several factors – urgency in care plan, shock, involvement of several care teams, etc. This can hinder "quick" understanding of the details of treatment plans, as well as delay the expected consent. Patient may utter words such as: "I'm tired…" or, "…Can I think about it…" The presence of spiritual care can serve as a "bridge" by helping patient and/or family process the information received and to help navigate the way forward in the care plan. The state of mind, family dynamics and other important issues in the patient's life can contribute to her readiness or unpreparedness for care plan. Needless to say that the patient might intentionally delay his or her cooperation with the care team for the reason of fear and uncertainty! Sitting with patients in their moments of dilemma can help restore hope and assurance. It can, consequently, reduce length of hospital stay and its consequent medical bills.

Trigger #13: **Voiced or Perceived Dilemma on plan of care**

- ◈ Patient needs clarification for faith reasons.
- ◈ He or she might just need someone with whom to share their "fears" or dilemmas – may be in need of validation, or language consistent with faith-belief, etc.

It is not unusual to find oneself at a crossroad, even in the course of ordinary events of life. Such can also happen in critical moments like hospitalization. Clinicians often may wonder why a patient or family member would delay or hesitate in giving consent to a "necessary" procedure/surgery. Patient's delayed or refused consent may not be tantamount to misunderstanding the benefits of the prescribed procedure or surgery. Yet, a patient's dilemma can truly, sometimes, slow down the proposed medical action plan. The patient might simply need clarification to know if a plan of care is consistent with his/her faith tradition. He or she might just need someone with whom to share his / her "fears" or dilemmas, or may be in need of validation, or assurance that it is consistent with faith-belief, etc. Rather than engage in "arm-twisting" as perceived and voiced by some patients, the clinical care provider can get the same patient's consent, in a timely fashion, when other professional disciplines are consulted. The chaplain, for instance, may possibly bring hope where there's fear and anxiety, reassurance where there's doubt and uncertainty, comfort to replace gloominess, encouragement to fortify a tired and weary will, and, validation when the voice and concern seems not to be heard.

One of my patients once said: "I need to understand step one before you take me to step two. I'd liked to proceed step by step." And I asked: "What would be step one for you, Mr. T?" He replied: "I need to discuss with the physician and understand the purpose of the surgery before anyone seeks my signature on the consent forms." The conclusion of the encounter was an informative meeting, facilitated by myself, that enabled the attending physician to attend to the patient's concerns and questions, including fears and clarifications. Then I asked: "Is the first step satisfied, Mr. T?" It was a resounding "Yes!" Do I need to say that the consent was given without further delay? In the affirmative!

Trigger #14: **Death or its imminence**

◈ Loss of a patient

- Support for bereaved family;

- Support for unit's associate (if so affected).

- Associate's loss of a family member, friend, etc that might affect his/her disposition at work.

- Spiritual Care services are for patients, families, and care-providers (associates).

Chaplains receive the most calls for this reason – deaths on nursing units. As a matter of fact, clinicians often consider calling the pastoral / spiritual care department as soon as death occurs. My work relationship with nurses and doctors over the years reveals that some believe chaplains should be called "only" when death occurs, for the purpose of prayers/ rituals, comfort to the family and for their work to continue. While some "unintentionally," I suppose, ignores several other important reasons for chaplains' consult, they may remember at the 11:59:59-hour.

It suffices to say that this is but one of several roles of chaplains in the hospital or any care facility. When death occurs or is about to occur, a chaplain's presence can be comforting to the dying and/or family members present. It may be appropriate to honor the deceased or the dying with accustomed religious rituals such as Anointing of the Sick, Last Rites for the dying, Prayer for the dead, Final Commendation, Prayer for family members, significant rituals, and so on. This can be comforting to those present.

Chapter Seven

Care for the Care-Providers
Wellness of the "Desert Community"

One person caring about another represents life's greatest value!
- Jim Rohn

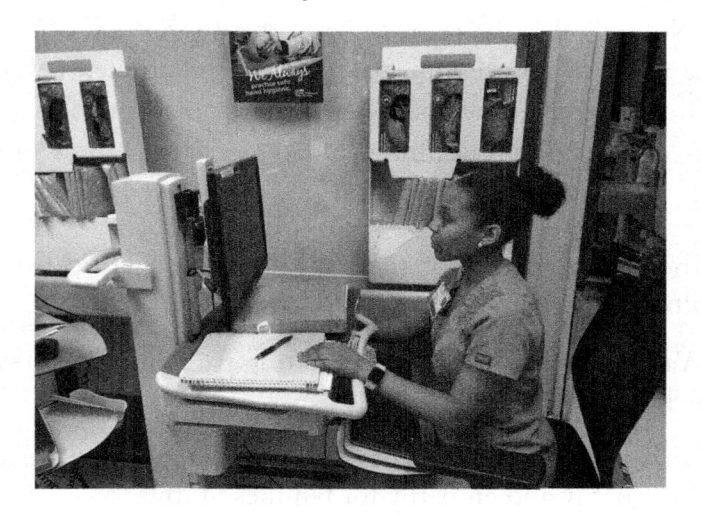

Objective

❖ To establish an awareness of spiritual care needs for clinicians

Care for Care Providers
Wellness for Clinicians

Listen to this: "The expectation that we [doctors and nurses] can be immersed in suffering and loss daily and not be touched by it is as unrealistic as expecting to be able to walk through water without getting wet. This sort of denial is no small matter."[88] Hearing this from the horse's mouth cannot be better expressed as Dr. Remen succinctly expressed the main preoccupation of this section of the book. To minimize the importance of care for clinicians – care providers – or accord it a total neglect will be to live in an absolute unrealistic professional world, to say the least. It will be a total disservice to those who use plunge their entire being to caring for others and who deserve to receive what they, in turn, give to others. To plow through understanding the need for caring for clinicians, it may be important to rhetorically ask, 'Why Spiritual Care for Clinicians?' In some of the lectures I have facilitated for Resident Doctors, someone once asked: "…and who cares for us?" What a realistic question! Yes, who provides support for the care providers as to ensuring their continued wellness! Not only it is the right thing to do, it is a NECESSARY care to provide so as to ensure and guarantee the continued **safety of the patients** being served. The following reasons may provide additional justifiable reasons to seek wellness and integral wholeness of the care providers:

- The critical nature of their work –sudden critical or chronic illness leading to sudden death, etc.
- Watching people suffer excruciating pain and agony – terminal sickness, etc.
- Losing patients with whom they've developed work relationship – sympathy and empathy for families in "misery."
- Death of a co-worker, colleague
- Hospital systemic structure – high acuity
- "Work-continues-syndrome"
- Staffing shortages/personnel
- Other work-related issues and concerns
- One's own family issues, life peculiar situations

It is crucial for clinical staff or associates to achieve balance in and between their professional and personal lives. The spiritual/pastoral care providers seek to empathize with patients and families, as they deal with critical diagnoses, treatment plans, unexpected downturns, poor prognoses, natal/fetal demise, etc. Their feelings are extremely important and should not be ignored. Spiritual care service can help at such moments for care providers like them. The non-judgmental spiritual care, hence, is not concerned with their religious practices but in their own unique and integral relationships among the "worlds" that define THEM and the care THEY provide. It is pertinent to say that 'Spiritual Care' begins with reflecting on one's own spiritual nature or journey, enabling the care provider to give from her or his arsenal of treasure. In brief, spiritual care is a support system to help process and understand the reality of human mortality and the limitation of human technology. It also helps to provide support as the care provider deal with the illness or loss of a co-worker, a friend or a colleague. Overall, the presence and the professional assistance of a chaplain can help bring some closure to grief and loss that the care provider may be experiencing, thereby initiating healing process and the restoration of peace and acceptance.

They may need to discuss any of these situations with someone. In bringing clinicians and associates the skills to address the spiritual needs of their patients, they have to start with themselves reflecting on their own spiritual nature and journey. It is giving from one's treasure.

For selfless and caring physicians and nurses, spiritual care is a support system to help process the loss of a dear patient; the pain and grief they share with families in grief, the frustrations, disappointments and feelings of helplessness especially in their hopeful desire to save lives.

Spiritual care provides the service for this realization.

Spiritual Wellness Neglect – A Costly Price!

Straight to the point – neglect of integral, holistic wellness of the care providers (clinicians) may inadvertently compromise patient safety! Quality of patient care is greatly at risk! This is a costly price for any hospitals or health care centers to pay. Neglect, in this sense, means to 'disregard' or 'ignore' or 'undermine' the necessity of caring for one's own spiritual need or well-being. That is, the care provider stands the risk of losing grip of his or her wholeness whenever the spiritual wellness is fractured. It is crucial to remember that the conceptual understanding of spiritual care or wellness in this book is consistent, not necessarily about how religiously devoted, but how attentive an individual is to gaining strength, rejuvenation, and invigoration from what gives him or her meaning in life. Mauk & Schmidt write to substantiate the need for spiritual well-being and also warn against spiritual neglect:

- Clinicians and other hospital staff need to be able to replenish mental, spiritual as well as physical energy thereby restoring personal energy as they deliver exceptional patient care.
- The burden of compassionate care-giving can become overwhelming.
- An overwhelmed care provider is at risk for caregiver fatigue.
- Clinicians may suffer effects at various levels of caregiver fatigue, including **burnout** and **compassion fatigue,** both involving the depletion of energy.
- A protracted level of caregiver fatigue – burnout and/or compassion fatigue – can hinder the quality of service to patients and families, and also compromise patient safety goals.
- The myriad of consequences of fatigue include:
  - Reduction of skilful anticipation and patient safety.
  - Diminished judgment, degraded decision-making, slowed reaction time and lack of concentration.
  - Absenteeism.
  - Clinical errors, failure to rescue, falling asleep when driving.
  - Decreased quality of interaction with colleagues and patients.
  - Nurses' fatigue is one of the top three causes of drug errors identified by nurses, along with physician's handwriting and nurses' distraction.[89]

As it relates to patients' safety and excellent practice of medicine, it is important to draw upon statistics that show the correlation between fractured wholeness and professional malpractice that could result in fatal, or sometimes irreversible, damage or loss to patients and their loved ones:

- ❖ 16.5% of the nurses in a study by Deans (2005) identified fatigue as a cause of medication errors.
- ❖ Of 686 nurses surveyed by AORN (Association of Registered Nurses), 58% felt unsafe while providing patient care.
- ❖ 13% stated they had made patient care mistakes because of fatigue.
- ❖ 38% reported fatigue-related near errors.[90]

Spiritual wellness and healthy caregiver can deliver safe care!

Considering these significant numbers and the possible compromise of patient safety, it is therefore necessary to understand what fatigue is. But remember, spiritual wellness and healthy caregivers can ensure, improve and deliver a safe care environment.

Caregiver Fatigue

- ❖ **Fatigue is** an overwhelming, debilitating and sustained sense of exhaustion that decreases one's ability to carry out daily activities, including the ability to work effectively and to function at one's usual level in family or social roles.
- ❖ **Burnout** results from stress and psychological strain on the job. Burnout creates nurse "silencing responses" to client suffering which prevents connection (Baranowsky, 2002).[91] It is very fascinating to note how Dr. Remen links "grieving and healing" to burnout. She asserts, "Protecting ourselves [doctors and nurses] from loss rather than grieving and healing our losses is one of the major causes of burnout."[92] Underscoring the importance of grieve as a therapeutic response to "burn out" syndrome, Remen

asserts that, "You grieve because it's of help to you. It enables you to go forward after loss. It heals you so that you are able to love again."[93]

◈ **Compassion Fatigue** is a mild or severe depletion of mental, psychological, or even physical energy such that it adversely affects the care provider's ability to provide effective care filled with empathy, patience, compassion, and love. For VanderZyl, compassion fatigue is a malaise of the spirit that results in a decreased capacity to care or the capacity to be filled with loving-kindness, patience, humility, and altruism. It should be noted that this all-encompassing physical, mental, social, and spiritual exhaustion often develop gradually, from weeks spanning through years.[94] Severe compassion fatigue may compromise all that good care stands for – safe, quality, efficient, and effective patient care.

Care must be taken that a professional care provider does not reach a point whereby the individual becomes emotionally numb or feels "nothing" in showing compassion and patience when providing care. It is worth quoting what some burnt-out professionals shared with Dr. Remen: "…I don't care anymore. Terrible things happen in front of me and I feel nothing." Contrary to the "On to the next" work syndrome at most hospitals, it is crucial to note that, such imbibed professional disposition "is a denial of a common humanity, an assertion that someone can die in front of us without touching us. It is a rejection of wholeness, of a human connection that is fundamental."[95]

Symptoms of Burnout and Caregiver Fatigue[96]

SYMPTOMS OF BURNOUT	SYMPTOMS OF CAREGIVER FATIGUE
Loss of compassion	Physical exhaustion
Listlessness	Sleep difficulty

Boredom	Physical symptoms (e.g. headaches or gastrointestinal symptoms)
Discouragement	Alcohol, drug, or food abuse
Impatience	Anger
Alienation	Blaming
Cynicism	Hopelessness
Negativism	Low self-esteem
Detachment	Decreased joy
Depression	Depression
	Workaholism

Box 2: Self-Assessment: Answer "yes" or "no" to the following nine statements[97]

Personal concerns commonly intrude on my professional role.	Yes	No
My colleagues seem to lack understanding	Yes	No
I find even small changes enormously draining	Yes	No
I can't seem to recover quickly after association with trauma	Yes	No
Association with trauma affects me very deeply	Yes	No
My patients' stress affects me deeply	Yes	No
I have lost my sense of hopefulness	Yes	No
I feel vulnerable all the time	Yes	No
I feel overwhelmed by unfinished personal business	Yes	No

Scale: Answering "yes" to four or more questions may indicate that you're suffering from or the risk of compassion fatigue is imminent.

Practical Suggestions

Tools and Tips: Based on your answers to Box 2 and perceivable symptoms in Box 1:

- ❖ Reflect and write down practical suggestions or action-plans geared toward spiritual self care, such as debrief, vacation, retreat (spiritual rejuvenation), a listening presence/chat with a chaplain, a pastor, a spiritual leader, a mentor, a confidant/friend, etc. **DO NOT** ignore as this may be detrimental to self and to the patients being cared for!

The underlying importance of this exercise is the realization that a healthy self is a good caring self! As research and studies have shown, patients will be safer in the hands of care-providers when they operate in a sound mind and integral wholeness. Hence, it should be noted that having completed the self-assessment and answering "yes" to four or more questions in the self-assessment box, you may be suffering from or be on the verge of compassion and caregiver fatigue. Then, the question is: What am I to do? Self-care!!! Holistic healing is a need not just for patients, but also for clinicians, other healthcare workers, and caregivers in general.

Chapter Eight

Spiritual Care for Cancer Patients

"Most of us have far more courage than we ever dreamed we possessed."
-*Dale Carnegie*

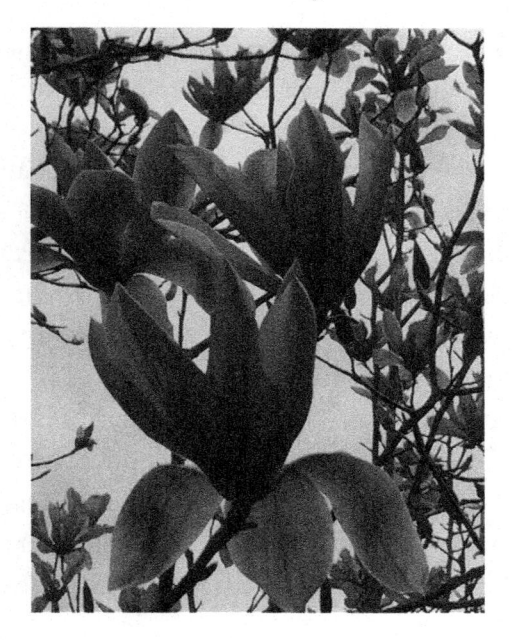

Objectives: The objectives in this chapter shall include:

- ❖ Brief insight into Malignant Neoplasms (Cancer) as a Killer Disease
- ❖ Understand Spiritual Assessments for Cancer Patients

Patients come to the hospital for different reasons – some, as a result of a conscious and willful decision for varied purposes, and some, for emergency reasons. Whatever reason brings a patient to the hospital, willful or not, it is most certainly true that a hospital visit is perceived as 'what I have to do because..." It is never a picnic ground! And it is never a facility, no matter what grandeur and magnificence the architectural design may reflect which anyone longs to visit. It becomes a truly scary place when a patient, on the first day, receives a life-changing result of a biopsy and it turns out to be malignant cancer! The mind quickly captures, perhaps, the reality of repeated hospital visits, among other legitimate concerns.

Among World's Top 10 killer diseases, Malignant Neoplasms ranked #4. Records show that 12.49% of annual worldwide deaths are caused by Malignant Neoplasms. Malignant Neoplasms is the medical term for 'cancer.' In 2007, 7.6 million people died from cancer. It is a class of disease in which a group of cells display uncontrolled growth, invasion and sometimes metastasis (spread to other locations in the body via lymph or blood).[98]

Steven Reinberg, in his article "Cancer Killed Almost 8 Million Worldwide in 2007" writes: "Cancer continues to cut a deadly swath across the globe, with the American Cancer Society reporting 12 million new cases of malignancy diagnosed worldwide in 2007, with 7.6 million people dying from the disease."[99] In fact, the World Health Organization (WHO) states, according to the statistics published in 2009 about cancer worldwide, that cancer is a "leading cause of death worldwide. It accounted for 7.4 million deaths (around 13% of all deaths) in 2004..."[100] Patients that are diagnosed of malignant neoplasms thus deserve more than a chapter in this book, not only because cancer is ranked as the fourth killer disease, but even more important such patients may soon embark upon a "beginning-of-the-end" life journey. According to the National Cancer Institute, there are over 200 types of cancers which can be categorized under: Carcinoma (Cancer that begins in the skin or in tissues that line or cover internal organs); Sarcoma (Cancer that begins in bone, cartilage, fat, muscle, blood vessels, or other connective or supportive tissue); Leukemia (Cancer that starts in blood-forming tissue such as the bone marrow and causes large numbers of abnormal blood cells to be produced and enter the blood); Lymphoma and myeloma (Cancers that begin in the cells of the immune system) and, Central nervous system cancers (Cancers that begin in the tissues of the brain and spinal cord). Not only do the scary types (and numbers) of cancer send shock waves through the nervous system of any human, but their incessant growth is also alarming. The World Health Organization (WHO) declared, in the 2009 general information about cancer, that "Deaths from cancer worldwide are projected to continue rising, with an estimated 12 million deaths in 2030."[101] Invariably, the world would witness an increase of 4.6 million deaths traceable to cancer as its primary causal agent. What a cause for worry! Human worry is not limited to the relentless growth rate (per stats) but the failure of 21st century science and the practice of Western medicine to curb the ravaging power of cancer from snatching its "victims" from the earth with indescribable pains – physical, emotional, and psychological.

It can be psychologically "depressive" when a patient, say a newly diagnosed cancer patient, thinks about the "death rate" vs. "survival rate" especially when the cancer is at its final stage – metastasis. Focusing on the United States, the National Cancer Institute (2010) brings the reality closer in its published statistical figures, showing projected new cases and consequent death rates:

Cancer type	Estimated new cases	Estimated deaths
Bladder	70,530	14,680
Breast (female-male)	207,090-1,970	39,840-390
Colon and rectal (combined)	142,570	51,370
Endometrial	43,470	7,950
Kidney (renal cell)	53,581	11,997
Leukemia	43,050	21,840
Lung (including bronchus)	222,520	157,300
Melanoma	68,130	8,700
Non-Hodgkin lymphoma	65,540	20,210
Pancreatic	43,140	36,800
Prostate	217,730	32,050
Thyroid	44,670	1,690

(Source: Medicinenet.com 2012)

Anthony Ade Akinlolu

When the Journey Begins: Spiritual Care for Cancer Patients

Physical strength is measured by what we can carry; Spiritual by what we can bear.
—*Author Unknown*

The journey truly begins when suspicion is translated into medical tests and the series of tests are confirmed, especially when the biopsy result returns as positive. The mind oscillates between polarities of rhetorical questions, worries, and concerns. Among the many *"whys?"* are: 'Why me?' 'What have I done?' An overview of one's life quickly comes in a flash as if to say, 'What could be responsible for this?' The questions of "Why?" and "What?" often find no tangible or sensible answer regardless of how many times such questions were asked. The deepest yearning of the human person, in the face of perceived storms in life, calls out to what transcends the physical – the *inner* person – to the spirit within.

In reaching out to the inner person, the spirit within, the individual initiates a support system that can provide the envisaged help and strength that the physical body would need along the journey it's about to begin. The newly diagnosed cancer patient as well as patients already engaged in the medical battle with cancer would most likely reach for spiritual pillars to support the pains, discomforts and pangs of chemotherapy, radiation treatments, and so on. Research shows that "both patients and family caregivers commonly rely on spirituality and religion to help them deal with serious physical illnesses, expressing a desire to have specific spiritual and religious needs and concerns acknowledged or addressed by medical staff..."[102] In fact, King and Bushwick, in a survey of hospital inpatients, "found that 77% of patients reported that physicians should take patients' spiritual needs into consideration, and 37% wanted physicians to address religious beliefs more frequently."[103] While, more specifically, "A large survey of cancer outpatients in New York City found that a slight majority felt it was appropriate for a physician to inquire about their religious beliefs and spiritual needs, although only 1% reported that this had occurred. Those who reported that spiritual needs were not being met gave lower ratings to quality of care ($P < .01$)

and reported lower satisfaction with care ($P < .01$)."[104] Bowie, Sydnor and Granot also reported that "A pilot study of 14 African American men with a history of prostate cancer found that most had discussed spirituality and religious beliefs with their physicians; they expressed a desire for their doctors and clergy to be in contact with each other."[105] These research and survey facts underscore the relevance of spiritual care as a great support system for cancer patients – in/outpatients.

Spiritual Assessment for Cancer Patients

Having established the importance of spiritual care in the overall care plan for cancer patients, it is absolutely necessary for care providers to evaluate or appraise the spiritual needs of the patient. It goes without saying, as stated in chapter four, that "in order to assess spirituality, it is important for the clinicians to have some self-awareness of their own spirituality, to be able to care for their own spiritual needs, to establish a good relationship with the patient, and to time the discussion appropriately."[106] Bartel (2004), writing on the assessment of spiritual pain, affirms that it depends, "as much upon the spirituality of the caregiver, and upon their capacity for contemplation, for close listening, to narrative, for intuition, and for discernment, as it will upon the results of any neatly developed questionnaire." Puchalski's credible work "Spiritual Assessment in Clinical Practice" has tremendously contributed to the proficiency of chaplains' training and/or service. The *Assessment Tool* can, undoubtedly, provide invaluable adeptness into providing spiritual care for cancer patients. Because of its efficiency in a comprehensive evaluation of spiritual care need of the care-seeker, it shall be adopted in this work as a *Spiritual Care Assessment Tool* for cancer patients.

SPIRITUAL ASSESSMENT TOOL

A spiritual assessment tool has gained some prominence among spiritual caregivers as well as care-providers in hospitals, hospice or palliative care communities. In order to make conversation with patients concise, more friendly, and information-enriching, some sets of important spiritual inquiries are built into acronyms to assist physicians, nurses, care-providers and chaplains to assess spiritual dimensions of their patients in order to meet such spiritual needs. It is important to mention that these spiritual assessment tools can be used for all inpatients or home-service based patients, and not just cancer patients, even though it is discussed under this chapter. There are few of such Spiritual Assessment Tools. First, there is the SPIRIT developed by Ambuel B. and D.E. Weissman. SPIRIT:

- ❖ S – Spiritual belief system
- ❖ P – Personal spirituality
- ❖ I – Integration with a spiritual community
- ❖ R – Ritualized practice and restrictions
- ❖ I – Implications for medical care
- ❖ T- Terminal event planning.

Secondly, Christina Pulchalski developed a spiritual assessment tool, FICA an **acronym,** which can be used to remember what to ask in a spiritual care conversation with the patient or the care-seeker: ***FICA*** [107]

- ❖ **F:** Faith or Beliefs
- ❖ **I:** Importance and Influence
- ❖ **C:** Community
- ❖ **A:** Address or Application

F: "What do you believe in that gives meaning to your life? Do you consider yourself to be a religious or spiritual person?" Both religious and spiritual are used, Hallenbeck expatiates, because individuals may relate to one and may even take offense at the other. This further substantiates the initial assertion we made at the beginning (chapter one) about the clear distinction that exists between 'religiosity' and 'spirituality.'

I: "How important is your faith (or religion or spirituality) to you?" Just hearing that the person is spiritual or a member of a particular religion tells you little. How important is this? How is it crucial? There is a big difference between a Catholic who has not been to Mass since childhood and one who goes to Mass daily. No doubt, the latter would appreciate daily Communion (if able to eat) while hospitalized.

C: "Are you part of a religious or spiritual community?" Particularly for those who participate in an organized religion, community is often a central part of their spiritual and social experience. It is not uncommon that just when this community becomes most important, as death approaches, as stated earlier, the individual is cut off from that community because of illness and caregiving needs.

A: "How would you like me to address these issues in your healthcare?" "How might this matter apply to your current situation?" "How can we assist you in your spiritual care?" Patients and families often feel better simply because they have been granted permission to share their beliefs. That you have inquired is usually considered as a sign of respect.

General recommendations when taking a spiritual history:

1. Consider spirituality as a potentially important component of every patient's physical well being and mental health.

2. Address spirituality at each complete physical exam and continue addressing it at follow-up visits if appropriate. In patient care, spirituality is an on-going issue.

3. Respect a patient's privacy regarding spiritual beliefs; don't impose your beliefs on others.

4. Make referrals to chaplains, spiritual directors or community resources as appropriate.

5. Be aware that your own spiritual beliefs will help you personally

and will overflow into your encounters with those for whom you care to make the doctor-patient encounter a more humanistic one (Puchalski, 1999).

Sounding a cautionary note on physicians *vs.* spirituality, James Hallenbeck, physician, said in his book "Palliative Care Perspectives" that "it is not about you, it is about the patient and family." Addressing clinicians in training, he also posited "In teaching spirituality as a component of a broader palliative care curriculum, it is not what I, the teacher, believes or you, the learner, believes that is most important. It is about acquiring skills necessary to address the spiritual needs of patients and families, period."[108]

Karen Skalla (2005), working among Spiritual Care Special Interest Group (SIG) project for Oncology Nursing Society, offered some sample questions that might be helpful for care providers, physicians, nurses, chaplains, and others, when providing care for cancer patients:

- What things do you enjoy doing? Are you doing them now?
- Where does your sense of what to do come from?
- Do you have someone you talk to for [spiritual/religious] guidance [matters]?
- What gives your life meaning?
- What sustains you during difficult times?
- What do you hope for?
- Are you part of a religious or spiritual community? Is it a source of support? In what ways?
- What aspects of your religion/spirituality would you like me to keep in mind as I care for you?
- Does your religious or spiritual belief influence the way you look at your disease and the way you think about your health?
- As we plan for your care, how does your faith impact your decisions?[109]

Research demonstrates that spiritual needs vary as the individual seeks to make sense of the diagnosis, treatment, learning to live as a survivor, recurrence of disease, and end-of-life (Halstead & Hull, 2001; Taylor, 2000).

Spiritual Issues for Cancer Patients

"To love means loving the unlovable.
To forgive means pardoning the unpardonable.
Faith means believing the unbelievable.
Hope means hoping when everything seems hopeless."
—Gilbert Keith Chesterton

As said earlier in this chapter, hospitalization experience for cancer patients is not just a matter of an in-and-out routine hospital visit, nor is it a one-time visit purposed for curative or corrective medical intervention. Each visit carries with it the heaviness of dealing with "CANCER" in all its ramification and intensity. Hence, it is pertinent to tailor ALL CARES according to the special needs of oncology patients. Halstead and Taylor identified seven essential spiritual issues for cancer patients in their Spiritual Care Special Interest Group Toolkit project (2005). These are appropriate issues that I have also noticed in the course of my pastoral and spiritual care work at four different hospitals over an eight-year period. It suffices to say that these issues can also be appropriately applied to other hospitalized patients or any care-seeker; however, they truly capture the hemisphere of care that is appropriate for each and every cancer patient in his or her peculiar health ordeal. These seven spiritual issues will be appropriately adapted in this book. These issues are:

- ❖ Connecting
- ❖ Meaning and purpose in life
- ❖ Faith
- ❖ Forgiveness

- ❖ Hope
- ❖ Suffering
- ❖ End of Life

Connecting

Spiritual health is manifested when one experiences harmonious connections internally, with other persons and with nature, and with the cosmos and its Creator (Taylor, 2002; Goldberg, 1998). It is through our relationships with others that we can fully understand ourselves and nurture our spirituality (Burkhardt & Nagai-Jacobson, 2002).[110] According to Halstead and Taylor, facilitating connection is enabled as the nurse approaches the patient non-judgmentally and honestly. As trust develops – that is, interpersonal relationship – the nurse begins to assess the patient's relationship with God, a Higher Power, or nature – transpersonal relationship.[111] – (Halstead and Taylor, 2005). The patient, therefore, will be better supported with courage and strength, first from within the 'self' and then, from the immediate care providers. Connecting – through the immediate care providers – is not limited to the attending physician or nurse but also involves connecting with support groups representing similar health challenges. Experience has shown that there is a great strength derivable from group identification – moral strength, psychological encouragement, spiritual support, and physical fortification. "Connecting," Halstead and Taylor further suggest, "would involve providing the patients with relevant brochures; spiritual resource materials, intentional visits from chaplains or community clergy, prayers, and spiritual counseling." All these will be productive when done in attentive and responsive listening. The focus of this issue – connecting – is unflinching assurance and reassurance for the patient that "I am not alone."

Case Study: From "When God and Cancer Meet" by L. Ebb:

When I was in the hospital after my cancer surgery, a friend came into my room and told me God was going to teach me great things through this trial. I wanted to take the IV out of my arm, stab it in hers, and tell her, "You get in bed and learn great things from God, because I don't want to learn this way." The first person to really give me hope was a woman named Pat who came up to me after my first hospital cancer-support group meeting, put her arm around me, walked me to my car, and told me I would make it through my chemotherapy. Do you know why I believed her? I believed her because she sported a brightly colored scarf on her head, still bald from chemotherapy. I knew that she knew because she has been there. Now my life is filled with cancer survivors because I've spent the intervening years both as a volunteer cancer-support group facilitator and as an employed patient advocate in my oncologist's office. I have held the hands of hundreds of people with cancer, listened to the fears in their hearts, and seen what gave them hope. I know that cancer patients and their caregivers are longing for encouragement as they try to make sense of what might seem like senseless suffering. It is my prayer to bring you that encouragement.[112]

Practical Ways for Clinicians to Connect:

Writing under the subtitle "The Gift of Healing" in her Book, *Kitchen Table Wisdom*, which I have quoted previously in this book, Dr. Remen shared: "For a long time, I had carried the belief that as a physician my love didn't matter and the only thing of value I had to offer was my knowledge and skill. My training had argued me out of my truth." Here is the heart of her message: "Medicine is as close to love as it is to science, and its relationships matter even at the edge of life itself."[113] Love connects the physician to the patient, the care provider to the care receiver, far beyond the potency of the pills and the Ivs and the chemo! Love, imbued with compassion, penetrates to the entire fabrics of the patient, sedates all pains and worries beyond telling, lulls unpleasant regiments of the seemingly long road to cure, if at all possible. Straight from his heart, a patient shared with a group of people with cancer: "My doctor's love is as important to me as his chemotherapy, but he does not know."[114]

Cancer patients have described connectedness as a requisite to, and an important aspect of, nurse-provided spiritual care (Taylor, 2003).[115] A qualitative study of 28 cancer patients and family caregivers found that ways connectedness was desired included having the nurse or physician:

- Show kindness and respect (e.g., a smile, being nice, addressing person respectfully)

- Listen and talk (even "simple conversations" as one informant put it)

- Praying (privately for or with the client)

- Be authentic or genuine

- Be physically present (e.g., "be there when I need it" or "just stay for a few minutes")

- Relate to clients with symmetry, as partners or fellow humans (e.g., "show a personal interest, [client] not be a number").[116]

From the above six practical ways to connect, as outlined by Halstead and Taylor, oncology nurses as well as care providers for hospitalized patients are being reminded of the essential ingredients of care. This represents a care model that can facilitate holistic care for patients. However, as identified in the Spiritual Care Special Interest Group (SIG) project by Halstead and Taylor, it is important to point out some dispositions and professional conducts that could obstruct effective *connecting* between a patient and the care-provider (nurse or physician), called **barriers to connection:**

- Changing subjects during conversation with clients

- Avoiding topics that are uncomfortable for the nurse

- Providing pat answers

- Minimizing client distress (e.g., "It'll get better")

- Being sarcastic (i.e., mutedly angry) with clients

- Faking interest in listening

- Boredom with client interactions
- Fearing what client will say
- Fearing you will be unable to help (Halstead and Taylor, 2005)

Meaning and Purpose

Spirituality provides meaning to life, and meaning provides purpose when all that seems to remain in times of serious illness is personal identity and relationships (Tarumi, 2003).[117] Illness has the capacity to break down self-concept and remodel one's perspective on life, relationships and role. This necessitates reconstruction of life's purpose and meaning within the context of the experience. A life-threatening illness may force one to reassess beliefs regarding meaning, spirituality, life purpose and relationships, which may engender positive changes (Caron, 2005).[118] As discussed earlier in chapter two, when we discussed 'change' as one of the four effects of hospitalization, it is not unusual that the experience of hospitalization, especially the medical crisis of cancer, can invoke an ardent search for a sense of meaning and relevancy in their lives (Rumbold, 2003).[119] The journey and the battle for life can exhume all existential, temporal and spiritual, objects or beings that give meaning to the patient's life and that can possibly answer some of the innumerable rhetorical questions thrust at his or her purpose in life. It is also reasonable to accept that individual's level of endurance or tolerance is fortified depending on how much meaning he or she makes out of his or her ordeal experience. Viktor Frankl captured the essence of this when he wrote: "Man is not destroyed by suffering; he is destroyed by suffering without meaning" (1984).[120] Meaning, Caron opines, provides a reference point within which to face the threat of depression and despair surrounding end of life. The true pole that sustains a person's life in the face of hopelessness is the "pole of meaning" – even the tiniest filament of meaning. When the 'dot' of meaning and purpose is lost, the human mind expresses such thoughts as 'Why am I living?' Or, 'There's nothing to live for!' The more these or similar thoughts linger, the more the spiritual, psychological and emotional shock-absorbers are broken down.

Barriers to finding meaning

Caron (2005) identifies some roadblocks to successful search for meaning amidst the travails of life:

- Initial reluctance to engage in spiritual support because the individual does not consider him/herself religious.
- Lack of openness and reluctance to savor family support, group support, etc.
- Spiritual distress, rejection and/or denial of medical diagnosis.
- Disbelief, anger and frustration surrounding the seemingly long tunnel of illness.
- Lack of an existing framework within which to place meaning on the present challenges.
- Since spiritual beliefs assist facilitation of clarity regarding meaning in suffering and illness, lack of a construct within which to interpret life events and assign meaning to them may leave an individual with a sense of being adrift without purpose or hope.
- Byock (1996) purports that end of life presents a developmental stage through which one must progress in order to complete the dying process. This progression requires a reframing of meaning. If a person is unable or unwilling to complete this life stage, a barrier to finding richer meaning in the experience arises.

Faith

In the Letter to the Hebrews, the Christian Bible defines faith as "the assurance of things hoped for, the conviction of things not seen" (NRSV 11:1). This has been the fundamental "*definition*" of faith among scholars, great minds and theologians all through periods in history. Saint Thomas

Aquinas, distinguished religious and spiritual faith from human faith when he posited: "The faith of which we speak here is not the mere human faith by which we accept the testimony of men, but the faith by which we accept the revealed word of God. The object of faith is truth about God and the things that pertain to God."[121] The Angelic Doctor further distinguished faith from other things: first, the object of faith, he argued, is not something seen or sensed; nor, in itself, is this object grasped by the intellect (*intellectus*). Again, referencing the classical biblical definition that faith "is the evidence (or assurance) of things not seen" (Heb. 11:1). Secondly, the object of faith, according to St. Aquinas, cannot be the object of scientific knowledge (*scientia*). He concurred with St. Gregory who had opined (Hom. XXI in Ev.): "When a thing is manifest, it is the object, not of faith, but of perceiving."[122] St. Thomas Aquinas, in *Quaestiones disputatae de veritate*, q. 14, a. 2 ("On faith"), and further differentiated faith from all other things: "For by saying 'of things that are not apparent' one distinguishes faith from knowledge (*scientia*) and understanding (*intellectus*). Again, by saying 'the argument' one distinguishes faith from (i) opinion (*opinio*) and doubt (*dubitatio*), in which the mind is not convinced, i.e., not determined to some one thing, and also from (ii) all habits which are not cognitive. Again, by saying 'the substance of things to be hoped for' one distinguishes [faith in the proper sense] from (i) faith as it is commonly understood (*fides communiter accepta*), in accord with which we are said either to believe that which we strongly opine or to believe in the testimony of some human being, and also from (ii) prudence (*prudentia*) and the other cognitive habits, which are not ordered toward the things to hope for or which, if they are so ordered, are not such that a proper inception of the things to be hoped for comes to exist in us through them." In other words, faith is different from knowledge, understanding, opinion, and certainly does not permit doubt. Dionysius states "Faith is the enduring foundation of those who believe, putting them in the truth and putting the truth in them."[123]

St. Thomas Aquinas explains this in the same context as writer of the Letter to the Hebrews means: "the substance of things to be hoped for." Expatiating further, St. Thomas Aquinas posits that the cognition of truth is a thing to be hoped for, since beatitude is nothing other than a rejoicing in the truth, as Augustine says in the *Confessions*. And St. Augustine of Hippo says of faith, it is "a virtue by which things that are not seen are believed." It is reasonable to accept that human minds are not able to fathom the reality of life in its entirety. Also, the human intellect is not able to comprehend the totality of all existential entities, especially the invisible things. This fundamental truth goes further to admit that creatures and realities are not limited to what human eyes can behold or human minds can conceive. God's power manifested in creatures transcends human limitedness. As Dionysius expressed, then comes the gift of 'faith' as an "enduring foundation of those who believe." As a 'bridge' that connects the two worlds – visible and invisible, temporal and spiritual – faith holds as: "The unshakable and unquestionable hope in the things that have been announced to us by God and in the efficacy of our prayers." I believe this truth was rightly captured by Damascene.[124]

In different ways and to a varied level of magnitude, faith has been implored as a strong pillar that holds the entire human edifice in moments of crisis or as a bridge that ensures safe crossover from the stormy side to a gentle, refreshing pasture. Faith is a "universal phenomenon" (Fowler, 1981) characterized by a sense of coherence and meaning and purpose (O'Brien, 1999). Benson (1997) is correct to relate faith to expectancies about life, illness, spiritual concerns and so forth. Rather than seeing faith from a relaxation response perspective, it suffices to concur that faith possesses the inexplicable capacity to have "positive health benefits" (Benson, 1997). In the same trend, some renowned experts such as Koenig (1999), Pargament (1997), and Levin (1994) have researched the possible influence of religious practice, in relation to faith, on the healing process.

Benefits of Faith for Cancer Patients:
- Hope
- An avenue for giving and receiving prayer
- Connectedness
- Social support
- Peacefulness

- Self-confidence
- A sense of purpose
- Altruism
- Accessing a source of energy[125]

It is reasonable to add the following:

- Significant spiritual insight and interpretation for illness and suffering
- Increased level of coping with discomfort caused by frailty of the body – sickness
- Positive disposition toward caregivers and care-providers: such patients are characterized by admirable appreciation for every little care received regardless of paid service or not. Their disposition often includes a cheerful face, smiles, "thank yous!" etc.
- Openness to discussing the true and an unsugar-uncoated reality of their medical situation with their providers. Patients operating in this realm would often encourage "truthfulness," and "straightforwardness imbued with compassion" from their attending physicians.
- Patients appreciate including spiritual care in the overall plan of care. For instance, they ask for chaplain's visits, could ask prayer from and with their physicians and nurses, prefer their physicians and nurses to be positive in their conversations either per medical updates or outlining a medical plan of care. To be 'positive' is not tantamount to shielding or coating the truth about their health.

Faith Issues for Patients with Cancer:
- Guilt (Something I did caused my cancer; God is punishing me)
- Spiritual Distress (God abandoned me; God doesn't care about me anymore)
- Suffering (How can a loving God allow this to happen?)
- Anger at God[126]

Stages of Faith Development (Fowler, 1981)

Fowler believed that faith develops sequentially much as Piaget and Erikson described cognitive and social development. For Fowler, faith develops in community rather than in isolation. This holds true in the Christian faith tradition as attested by the words of Paul: "Thus faith comes from what is heard…" (Rom 10:17). Healthy faith develops in loving, caring contexts. The stages of Fowler's developmental theory are:

Age	Stage	Characteristics	Nursing Responsibilities
Infant	Primal Faith	Trust is a basis for faith development	Consistent, loving, respectful responses from caregivers
Early Childhood	Intuitive-Projective Faith	Impulsive, unconscious acceptance of what others tell them about faith	Telling faith based stories, modeling prayer, religious activities, simple repetitive songs
Childhood and Beyond*	Mythic-Literal Faith	Realistic, factual, black and white, no grey areas	Support participation in ritual; reading stories of faith; faith-based music
Adolescence and Beyond*	Synthetic-Cnventional Faith	Commonly accepted beliefs, view of God as a friend, but also begin to have doubts about God or spirituality	Calm acceptance of questions; listening; support participation in ritual
Young Adulthood and Beyond*	Individuative-Reflective	Unique, thoughtful, spiritual analysis leads to personal, self-directed faith	Acceptance of faith struggles; listening; support ritual
Early Midlife and Beyond	Conjunctive Faith	Connected; realizes that faith is personal and within but also transcendent; acceptance of mystical nature of faith	Teach contemplative prayer or meditation; Discuss ecumenism; Support ritual
Midlife and Beyond	Universalizing Faith	Holistic; faith becomes part of identity; consider actions in light of their values; faith drives actions rather than self	Allow time and privacy to practice contemplative prayer; few reach this stage—Mother Teresa, Gandhi, Billy Graham

Source: Based on information from Halstead & Nilssen, in press; Mauk & Schmidt, 2004; O'Brien, 1999; Taylor, 2002 as used by Halstead, M. (2005)

Forgiveness

In recent years there has been an explosion of scientific research related to the subject of forgiveness that provides tantalizing evidence of the power of forgiveness to enhance mental and physical health. Forgiveness is a cornerstone of most religious and spiritual traditions.[127] Forgiveness, as Azim Khamisa & Jillian Quinn pointed out in their article, plays a central role in Jewish, Christian, Islamic, Confucian, Buddhist, and Hindu thought. It is undoubtedly true, as Halstead pointed out, that patients, who are experiencing a life-changing event such as a cancer diagnosis, treatment, and survival, or death, often reevaluate personal and religious values. The need for forgiveness and reconciliation may weigh heavily on their minds (Halstead & Nilssen, in press; Mickley & Cowles, 2001). When patients are faced with the reality of mortality, there's every possibility that they might want to address previous life incidents. Hurts that eventually led to severed relationships and estrangement with family members or friends can become matters of urgent attention in their minds. That might involve the desire to reconnect with those from whom the individual patient has disconnected, for instance, parent and child or vice versa; among siblings, cousins or nephews, close or distant relations. This is because most people facing life-threatening illness want to depart the world in peace, and reconciliation and forgiveness is a pathway to such desired peace. Some patients do spend several hours of the day ruminating and wishing they could either see the estranged person in order to talk over things and possibly make peace. Some, though wronged, are prepared to forgive and let-go if only they can see the inflictor. Some are able to achieve this while others are not. However, it suffices for care providers to recognize the possibility of a cancer patient or anyone undergoing life-threatening illness to have "the need for forgiveness and reconciliation" staring at them in the face. Thus, forgiveness of self or others may be helpful in preventing or alleviating depression, anxiety, or other psychopathologies. Although forgiveness is a precedent for reconciliation, reconciliation does not always follow (Festa & Tuck, 2000). In this context it is important to remember Rhonda Britten's quotable quote: "Forgiveness is not a one-time-only event. It is a process." Patients dealing with life-threatening illness may be moving to initiate this process with every sense of urgency. According to Robert Enright, professor of human development at the University of Wisconsin at Madison, forgiveness researchers universally agree that forgiveness is not:

- ❖ Forgetting
- ❖ Condoning
- ❖ Excusing
- ❖ Trusting without reason
- ❖ Forgoing legal or financial reparation
- ❖ Reconciling if it would in any way endanger the victim's safety or health
- ❖ Forgoing justice—which in itself requires courage, an important expression of love.[128]

Forgiveness, as a spiritual value, dispels negative emotions while it opens the door for positive emotions, for self healing and greater concentration of the energy needed to focus on what should be first in the order of priority, here and now – healing of the self. Withholding forgiveness, either for self or for another person, makes holistic healing an upheaval task, if not unattainable. If withheld, it might become a destructive "psychological cancer."

Hope

Hope can be defined as the multidimensional, dynamic, and future-oriented expectation of achieving a positive outcome that has experiential, spiritual, rational and relational attributes that energize and provide a sense of freedom and resiliency (Felder, 2004). Cancer patients have identified hope as one of the most essential elements in their lives (Chapman & Pepler, 1998; Ballard, et al., 1997; Herth, 1990); hope and healthy spirituality are closely linked (Post-White, et al., 1996). Oncology nurses are in a unique position to inspire or nurture hope in our patients.

We can accomplish this by incorporating presence, touch, active listening, humor or a sense of lightheartedness, and spirituality into our practices (Poncar, 1994; Herth, 1990). We can further nurture hope by helping our patients establish meaningful support systems, affirming their worth as individuals, and helping them recall positive memories (Herth, 1990).

Clinicians and care providers have a responsibility to promote hope that is realistic. This can be accomplished by assisting patients in practicing reality surveillance, cognitive restructuring or reframing, values clarification, and setting realistic goals (Poncar, 1994; Herth, 1990; Miller, 1984).

Keeping the Flame of Hope Alive

It is imperative for clinicians to inspire hope among patients. Inspiring hope is not tantamount to "sugar-coating" realities surrounding the patient's illness and medical prognosis. It also is not raising "false hope" for the patient and family, by shielding them from the inevitable staring at them. One of my patients once told me, "Please, I don't want Dr. X here anymore…I'd appreciate another doctor other than him…he's not open with me, he seems to hide the truth…" The patient was one among many patients who had indicated to me, in the course of spiritual care service, that she would prefer her doctor to be "straightforward." I did include in her chart that the patient values "facts, honesty and medical truth." This is not to close, prematurely, any possible window of hope that could give meaning and relevance to today's sufferings and inconveniences that the patient is enduring. Similarly, as written by Felder (2005), clinicians should avoid hope-hindering practices which patients have identified as poor symptom management, the sense of isolation or abandonment, and the devaluation of personhood. Providing information in an honest, respectful, compassionate manner can increase levels of hope. Conversely, providing information in a disrespectful or cold manner, trivializing the situation, or giving discouraging medical facts without offering something to hold on to decrease levels of hope (Koopmeiners, et al., 1997; Herth, 1990). Hope may be all that is left for the patient to cling to and it would be damaging if this precious pearl, in the wake of crushing illness, is taken from the patient. It may also be part of the support mechanism that keeps the patient through each of the cancer treatments and possibly beyond. At the dawn of each day, as it were, the hope is renewed and the patient gear up for whatever the day holds. Orison Swett Marden (1850 – 1924), an American author and founder of Success Magazine, captured the truth and the reality about hope when he said: "There is no medicine like hope, no incentive so great, and no tonic so powerful as expectation of something tomorrow." Every patient, every cancer patient lives today in the hope for tomorrow!

Suffering

What is suffering? As many theoretical definitions abound for the concept of 'suffering,' so also will practical descriptions and/or definitions exist widely. Eifried (2005) pulled some resources that offer succinct description and definition to the subject under review. First, citing the practical experience of Cassell, a physician, who experientially defined 'suffering' as: "a distressful state induced by the possibility of losing one's sense of living as an integrated being" (1992).[129] Secondly, from a theoretical standpoint, Kahn and Steeves (1986), oncology nurses, opined that "suffering is experienced when some crucial aspect of one's self, being, or existence is threatened."[130] Rawlinson posits that "Suffering involves frustrated purposes and unrealized possibilities" (1986). If illness, deprivation, pain, or disability obstructs one's access to the world and constricts one's horizons, suffering occurs. Suffering is not necessary to find meaning, but even in the face of suffering, meaning is possible (Frankl, 1985). The suffering that a cancer patient endures seems to be peculiar. It is undoubtedly correct that patients undergo suffering and discomforts at different levels and magnitudes. In many cases, such sufferings, pains, and discomforts can be very momentary, for instance, the discomfort of general hospitalization, pains from post-surgery or medical procedure (after anesthesia's expiration), pains from needle-sticks, etc. When these medical events are over, there's every possibility that the individual resumes his or her normal course of life without any prolonged aftermath. The story seems to be different with cancer patients. From the moment when the individual receives his or her test results and the diagnosis is subsequently confirmed, perhaps through a second opinion, the mental agony begins, especially with a metastasized malignant tumor. Working with cancer patients truly reveals that the treatment options available, so far in the world of medicine, are such that the treatment plan can be in a series of which the aftermaths are nothing but excruciating pain. Such may include one or more of these: chemotherapy, radiation therapy, surgery, and transplantation. Sometimes, the drastic "change" in disposition of a cancer patient-in-treatment prior to chemotherapy, for instance, and post chemotherapy is really indescribable. It beggars description to an even greater extent when the stages of the chemo treatments begin to take their toll on the patient. All that might readily come to one's mind is 'suffering.' Why not? Some significant side effects of chemotherapy, for instance, would confirm this. Such include anemia, appetite change, bleeding problems, constipation, diarrhea, fatigue, hair loss (alopecia), infection, memory changes, swelling (fluid retention), mouth and throat changes, nausea and vomiting, nerve changes, pain, sexual and fertility changes in men, sexual and fertility changes in women, and, urination changes.[131] These possible side effects most often engender anxiety and fear of uncertain outcomes. This is why, as some cancer patients would say, there is more to deal with than the mouth can truly explain. Considering the enormity of what a cancer patient has to endure, patients need to be supported (Eifried, 2005; Lewis, 1982; &Taylor, 1993).

Suffering the deadly disease of cancerous tumor can also be complicated when a patient finds himself or herself on a seemingly "long" road, alone and abandoned by friends and family members. Mother Teresa of Calcutta captured it succinctly: "I have come to realize more and more that the greatest disease and the greatest suffering is to be unwanted, unloved, uncared for, to be shunned by everybody, to be just nobody." There is no doubt that a good support system can truly help to alleviate suffering and pain – physical, psychological, and spiritual. Nurses, physicians and other care providers can assist patients identified as having no family or friends or any visitor in days of hospitalization by sparing a few extra minutes to share some friendly conversations that can enliven the patient's spirit and dispel or reduce the already existing mood of loneliness and abandonment.

Nurses and physicians caring for oncology patients would be contributing to a viable healing environment as well as helping to ease sufferings if they demonstrate care imbued with empathy, care for the human person and not just the illness, concern about the patient's feelings here-and-now, staying with the patient and not above her, conversing and not just instructing, using the art of listening and not just talking-over, validating and not shutting-down. Perhaps, it doesn't take much to ease someone's pain – little words of encouragement, a little smile to cheer up, a human touch to shrink the gap and distance, enabling a patient to feel that my physician or nurse is 'here with me' and not just 'for me' thus maintaining a "compassionate presence" (Taylor, 1993).[132]

It is pertinent, as Eifried stated that nurses must not run from their feelings of helplessness in the presence of patient suffering. Nurses can assist patients to give voice to their suffering and expression to the ways that the suffering can be relieved (Eifried, 2005). Some useful resources are provided at the end of this chapter.

End-of-Life

The Christian sacred Scripture articulates the mortality of creatures when it states: "A time to be born, and a time to die; a time to plant, and a time to uproot the plant" (Eccl 3:2). That is, whatever has a beginning is sure to have an end, says the common wise saying. It is tantamount to saying that death is inevitable; transience is natural to all created beings, and every human person is born to die! As fundamental as this reality might be, yet it seems that human beings are still confounded as to when, where, or what would cause the inevitable. The possible causal agent may turn out to be cancer and its related complications when someone is diagnosed and started on the treatment plans – treatment without cure. At the confirmation of stage four cancer, part of what could possibly surface in the individual's world is end-of-life. There could be an eruption of past life events, a quick review of 'what must have caused this?' Or, some spontaneous rhetorical questions: 'Why me?' 'What did I do to deserve this?' In some cases, it may feel like receiving a "death sentence" as the oncologist presents to the patient an approximate length of his or her remaining days. This can be psychologically traumatizing as the person begins a "count down." This is the beginning of the end! All the above-discussed issues – spiritual issues for cancer patients – would congregate at the final bus stop – the domain of end-of-life. More than ever before, the patient needs love and support, not out of pity but as a matter of what he or she deserves from the community that loves and cares. As the patient grapples with the reality of human mortality, groping for meaning and purpose of life and existence, confronting the uncertainty of the world unknown, it behooves caregivers and/or care-providers to hold up gently the delicate pillars of life through words of reassurance, liberating words from guilt and regrets, upholding even the tiniest accomplishment or achievement of the patient, offering a positive outlook, and so on. More importantly, the patient needs the gift of presence from loved ones, as no one wants to die lonely. Loneliness, according to many experts, is not necessarily being alone but the perception of being alone and isolated. One of my patients once said: "I have many people come visit but I still feel lonely." And another patient shared: "I'm afraid because I don't know what lies ahead…what's on the other side." In other words, loneliness is not an absence of physical visitors. For someone approaching end-of-life, meaningful visits would be very helpful. It is important to engage the patient in such a manner that helps give credits to what they might be proud of as well as naming some possible regrets. Bronnie Ware, an Australian nurse who spent several years working in palliative care, caring for patients in the last twelve weeks of their lives, documented their dying revelations in a book entitled The Top Five Regrets of the Dying. These are the top five regrets of the dying, as witnessed by Ware:

- ◈ I wish I'd had the courage to live a life true to myself, not the life others expected of me.
- ◈ I wish I hadn't worked so hard.

- ❖ I wish I'd had the courage to express my feelings.
- ❖ I wish I had stayed in touch with my friends.
- ❖ I wish that I had let myself be happier.[133]

Could spouses or family members or caregivers be more courageous in engaging their dying loved one in some pertinent conversations: 'What are your happy moments?' 'What would you have loved to do differently?'

Chapter Nine

The Twilight
Faith Traditions in Death & Dying

To fear death, my friends, is only to think ourselves wise, without being wise: for it is to think that we know what we do not know. For anything that men can tell, death may be the greatest good that can happen to them: but they fear it as if they knew quite well that it was the greatest of evils. And what is this but that shameful ignorance of thinking that we know what we do not know?

–Socrates *(BC 469-BC 399)*

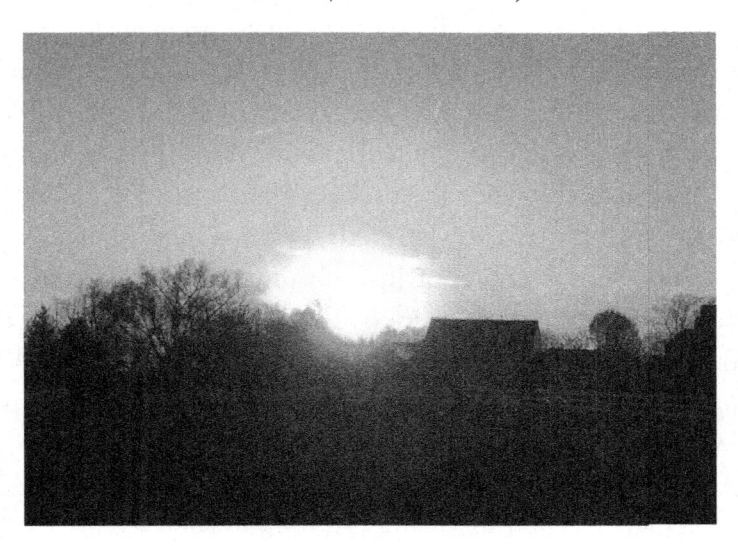

British poet and playwright, William Shakespeare (1564-1616) once said, "All that live must die, passing through nature to eternity." And the Christians' sacred Scripture warns: "There is an appointed time for everything, and a time for every affair under the heavens. A time to be born, and a time to die; a time to plant, and a time to uproot the plant" (Eccl 3: 1-2, NAB)! The rhythm of human existence, therefore, is built on 'time' – birth, living, and death. This complete human circle attests to the temporality of human beings, tall or short, black or white, fat or thin. Incidentally, just as the individual has no control as to where or when the life on earth begins, it is rarely possible to gain control of the 'time' for earthly departure, not speaking about violence to self. The departure, for some, arrives suddenly, due to accidental occurrence such as auto accident, travel mishaps (plane crash or ship capsizing), or domestic violence (gun shots, stabbings, intentional fire disaster, intentional poisoning, etc). For some, it may be just a one-time strike, leaving them no second chance. For still others, earthly departure is best described as 'the beginning of the end.' This is because, perhaps, the individual suffers an unexpectedly terminal illness such as stage 4 metastasized cancer, complications from chronic illness including multiple organ failure, and so on. For those whose earthly exit is preceded by "slow but gradual death," there is, at least, some chance to prepare for the final lap of their earthly existence. That is, they mostly stand the chance to evaluate and reevaluate their past and then engage the truth of their mortality in conscious preparation. They are able, for instance, to put their house in order, settle all scores (if possible), make peace and reconciliation with the Ultimate Divine, with people in their lives, and with themselves. There's the natural inclination to engage the spiritual self very strongly, perhaps more than ever before. The preparation, however, is not just within the dying person but also aided by caregivers and care providers. The pertinent questions are: 'How do I help you (the dying) journey peacefully to the other side?' 'What are the strengths and values in your spiritual beliefs that can help peaceful transition?'

These are legitimate concerns. Peaceful transition is desirable for anyone at the end of their lives. Understanding 'what to do' and 'how to respect' the religious beliefs of the dying person can be comforting to the dying as well as family members and other caregivers.

Death & Dying: Jewish Tradition

Jewish Faith Tradition: A Synoptic Overview

In North America today, the four main branches of Judaism are Orthodox, Conservative, Reform, and Reconstructionist. Within these denominations themselves, however, there is a great degree of variation in practice and observance.

Orthodoxy is the modern classification for the traditional section of Jewry that upholds the halakhic way of life as illustrated in a divinely ordained Torah. Halakha refers to the legal aspect of Judaism, and is also used to indicate a definitive ruling in any particular area of Jewish law.

Reform Judaism (also known as Liberal or Progressive Judaism) subjects religious law and customs to human judgment, attempting to differentiate between the facets of the Torah that are divine mandate and those that are specific to the time in which they were written.

Conservative Judaism developed mainly in the twentieth century as a reaction to Reform Judaism's liberalism. It sought to conserve tradition by applying new, historical methods of study within the boundaries of Jewish law to the mainstream of American society. It is the largest denomination of the four.

Reconstructionism is the most recent denomination within Judaism, and, rejecting the assertion that the Torah was given to Moses at Mount Sinai, views Judaism as a continual process of evolution, incorporating the inherited Jewish beliefs and traditions with the needs of the modern world. In addition to the four main branches, there are several other Jewish movements. **Jewish Renewal** is a trans-denominational movement grounded in Judaism's prophetic and mystical traditions. It seeks to restore the spiritual vitality of the 19th century Hasidic movement, yet like the Reconstructionist movement, believes that Judaism is an evolving religious civilization. Therefore, Jewish Renewal regards men and women as fully equal and welcomes homosexuals and converts.

Secular Humanistic Judaism is a movement that began in the 1960s which embraces "a human-centered philosophy that combines rational thinking with a celebration of Jewish culture and identity." In the Humanistic Jewish view, the focus is not on a relationship with God or religious ritual but in a belief that the "secular roots of Jewish life are as important as the religious ones." The emphasis is therefore placed on celebrating the Jewish *human* experience, and Jewish tradition, culture, ethics, values, and relationships (Jewish Outreach Institute, 2008).

It is crucial to mention that perspectives on life and death are essentially or fundamentally similar among these different groups in the Jewish tradition. However, it is important to know that these different branches exist and there may be possible peculiar customary practices, depending on the individual or group's tenets. Suffice it to say that this book will not attempt to uncover all intricacies, infinitesimal differences, and possible variations among the four branches that exist in Jewish tradition.

Common Perspectives of Jewish Tradition on Life, Death & Mourning

Perspective on Life

- ❖ Torah is the foundational basis of Jewish Law.
- ❖ In Judaism, life is valued above almost all else. The Talmud notes that all people are descended from a single person, thus taking a single life is like destroying an entire world, and saving a single life is like saving an entire world.
- ❖ Of the 613 commandments, only the prohibitions against murder, idolatry, incest and adultery are so important that they cannot be violated to save a life. Judaism not only permits, but often *requires* a person to violate the commandments if necessary

to save a life. A person who is extremely ill, for example, or a woman in labor, is not permitted to fast on Yom Kippur, because fasting at such a time would endanger the person's life. Doctors are permitted to answer emergency calls on the Sabbath, even though this may violate many Sabbath prohibitions. Abortions where necessary to save the life of a mother are mandatory (the unborn are not considered human life in Jewish law, thus the mother's human life overrides).

◆ Because life is so valuable, we are not permitted to do anything that may hasten death, not even to prevent suffering. Euthanasia, suicide, and assisted suicide are strictly forbidden by Jewish law. The *Talmud* states that you may not even move a dying person's arms if that would shorten his life.

◆ However, where death is imminent and certain, and the patient is suffering, Jewish law does permit one to cease artificially prolonging life. Thus, in certain circumstances, Jewish law permits "pulling the plug" or refusing extraordinary means of prolonging life.[134]

◆ Because the body belongs to God, Jews must seek both preventive and curative medical care and follow the experts' advice in preserving their health. The patient has the right to choose which regime to follow, as long as it fits within the rubric of Jewish law.

◆ With respect to critical care issues, the medical staff should ask the patient whether they want to consult their family members or their rabbi when filing out advance directives or in coming to a decision about what to do.

Determining Death

◆ The traditional criteria for death in Jewish tradition are cessation of breathing and heartbeat. Conservative rabbis have accepted brain death (including the brainstem) as fulfilling the traditional criteria of cessation of breathing and heartbeat.

◆ The strictest position restricts permission to withdraw or withhold treatment to situations for which doctors assume that the patient will die within 72 hours and has lost the swallowing reflex.

The Dying Process

- ❖ The Jewish tradition of never leaving the bedside of the dying is of immense value, not only to the dying person but also to family and friends.
- ❖ A dying Jew might request the presence of a rabbi at any time to go through the ceremony of *viddui* (confession) and to pray with the patient. This request should be honored, giving the patient and the rabbi peace and quiet to talk and pray together.

Death

In Judaism, death is not a tragedy, even when it occurs early in life or through unfortunate circumstances. Death is a natural process. Our deaths, like our lives, have meaning and are all part of G-d's plan. In addition, we have a firm belief in an afterlife, a world to come, where those who have lived a worthy life will be rewarded.

Mourning practices in Judaism are extensive, but they are not an expression of fear or distaste for death. Jewish practices relating to death and mourning have two purposes: to show respect for the dead (*kavod ha-met*), and to comfort the living (*nihum avelim*), who will miss the deceased.[135]

Care for the Dead: When Death Occurs

- ❖ After a person dies, the eyes are closed, the body is laid on the floor and covered, and candles are lit next to the body (live candles cannot be lit in the hospital; hence, the spiritual care department can be contacted for religious battery-powered candles). A candle may be placed near the head symbolic of the human soul and of God's eternal presence. *If death occurs on the Sabbath (sundown Friday through sundown Saturday)* **this should not be done.** As it is customary in most hospitals, if not all, a clean white sheet can be drawn to cover the entire body of the deceased including the face.

- ❖ The position of the body should be such that the feet face the doorway. The body should not be touched except to straighten the body if it is in an awkward position.

- ❖ The body is never left alone until after burial, as a sign of respect. The people who sit with the dead body are called *shomerim*, from the root *Shin-Mem-Resh*, meaning "guards" or "keepers."

- ❖ Respect for the dead body is a matter of paramount importance. For example, the *shomerim* may not eat, drink, or perform a commandment in the presence of the dead. To do so would be considered mocking the dead, because the dead can no longer do these things.

- ❖ Most communities have an organization to care for the dead, known as the *chevra kaddisha* (the holy society). These people are volunteers. Their work is considered extremely meritorious, because they are performing a service for someone who can never repay them.

- ❖ Autopsies in general are discouraged as desecration of the body. They are permitted, however, where it may save a life or where local law requires it. When autopsies must be performed, they should be minimally intrusive.

- ❖ The presence of a dead body is considered a source of ritual impurity. For this reason, a _kohein_ may not be in the presence of a corpse. People who have been in the presence of a body wash their hands before entering a home. This is to symbolically remove spiritual impurity, not physical uncleanness: it applies regardless of whether you have physically touched the body.

- ❖ In preparation for the burial, the body is thoroughly cleaned and wrapped in a simple, plain linen shroud. The sages decreed that both the dress of the body and the coffin should be simple, so that a poor person would not receive less honor in death than a rich person. The body is wrapped in a <u>tallit</u> with its *tzitzit* rendered invalid. The body is not embalmed, and no organs or fluids may be removed.

- The body must not be cremated. It must be buried in the earth. Coffins are not required, but if they are used, they must have holes drilled in them so the body comes in contact with the earth.

- The body is never displayed at funerals; open casket ceremonies are forbidden by Jewish law. According to Jewish law, exposing a body is considered disrespectful, because it allows not only friends, but also enemies to view the dead, mocking their helpless state.

- Jewish law requires that a tombstone be prepared, so that the deceased will not be forgotten and the grave will not be desecrated. It is customary in some communities to keep the tombstone veiled, or to delay in putting it up, until the end of the 12-month mourning period. The idea underlying this custom is that the dead will not be forgotten when they are being mourned every day. In communities where this custom is observed, there is generally a formal unveiling ceremony when the tombstone is revealed.[136]

Mourning

- Jewish mourning practices can be broken into several periods of decreasing intensity. These mourning periods allow the full expression of grief, while discouraging excesses of grief and allowing the mourner to gradually return to a normal life.

- When a close relative (parent, sibling, spouse or child) first hears of the death of a relative, it is traditional to express the initial grief by tearing one's clothing. The tear is made over the heart if the deceased is a parent, or over the right side of the chest for other relatives. This tearing of the clothing is referred to as *keriyah* (lit. "tearing"). The mourner recites the blessing describing G-d as "the true Judge," an acceptance of G-d's taking of the life of a relative.

- From the time of death to the burial, the mourner's sole responsibility is caring for the deceased and preparing for the burial. This period is known as *aninut*. During this time, the mourners are exempt from all positive commandments ("thou shalts"), because the preparations take first priority. This period usually lasts a day or two; Judaism requires prompt burial.

- During this *aninut* period, the family should be left alone and allowed the full expression of grief. Condolence calls or visits should not be made during this time.

- After the burial, a close relative, near neighbor or friend prepares the first meal for the mourners, the *se'udat havra'ah* (meal of condolence). This meal traditionally consists of eggs (a symbol of life) and bread. The meal is for the family only, not for visitors. After this time, condolence calls are permitted.[137]

- The next period of mourning known as *shiva* (seven, because it lasts seven days) shall not be discussed in this book, considering the target readership.

Death & Dying in the Tibetan Buddhist Tradition

Understanding Death in the Tibetan tradition:

There are two common meditations on death in the Tibetan tradition. The first looks at the certainty and imminence of death and what will be of benefit at the time of death, in order to motivate us to make the best use of our lives. The second is a simulation or rehearsal of the actual death process, which familiarizes us with death and takes away the fear of the unknown, thus allowing us to die skillfully. Traditionally, in Buddhist countries, one is also encouraged to go to a cemetery or burial ground to contemplate death and become familiar with this inevitable event.[138] As to the inevitability of death, the tradition holds the following:

- There is no possible way to escape death. No one ever has, not even Jesus, Buddha, etc. Of the current world population of over five billion people, almost none will be alive in 100 years time.

- ◈ Life has a definite, inflexible limit and each moment brings us closer to the finality of this life. We are dying from the moment we are born.

- ◈ Death comes in a moment and its time is unexpected. All that separates us from the next life is one breath.

The physiology of death revolves around changes in the winds, channels and drops. Death begins with the sequential dissolution of the winds associated with the four elements (earth, water, fire and air). "Earth" refers to the hard factors of the body such as bone, and the dissolution of the wind associated with it means that this wind is no longer capable of serving as a mount or basis for consciousness. As a consequence of its dissolution, the capacity of the wind associated with "water" (the fluid factors of the body) acts as a mount for consciousness becoming more manifest. The ceasing of this capacity in one element and its greater manifestation in another is called "dissolution" - it is not, therefore, a case of gross earth dissolving into water.

Simultaneously with the dissolution of the earth element, four other factors dissolve (see Chart 1), accompanied by external signs (generally visible to others) and an internal sign (the inner experience of the dying person). The same is repeated in serial order for the other three elements (see Charts 2-4), with corresponding external and internal signs.

The 8 Signs of Death in the Tibetan Buddhist Tradition

CHART 1: FIRST CYCLE OF SIMULTANEOUS DISSOLUTION		
Factor dissolving	**External sign**	**Internal sign**
earth element	body becomes very thin, limbs loose; sense that body is sinking under the earth	
aggregate of forms	limbs become smaller, body becomes weak and powerless	

basic mirror-like wisdom (our ordinary consciousness that clearly perceives many objects simultaneously)	sight becomes unclear and dark	appearance of mirages
eye sense	one cannot open or close eyes	
colors and shapes	luster of body diminishes; one's strength is consumed	

CHART 2: SECOND CYCLE OF SIMULTANEOUS DISSOLUTION

Factor dissolving	External sign	Internal sign
water element	saliva, sweat, urine, blood and regenerative fluid dry greatly	
aggregate of feelings (pleasure, pain and neutrality)	body consciousness can no longer experience the three types of feelings that accompany sense consciousnesses	
basic wisdom of equality (our ordinary consciousness mindful of pleasure, pain and neutral feelings as feelings)	one is no longer mindful of the feelings accompanying the mental consciousness	appearance of smoke
ear sense	one no longer hears external or internal sounds	
sounds	'ur' sound in ears no longer arises	

CHART 3: THIRD CYCLE OF SIMULTANEOUS DISSOLUTION

Factor dissolving	External sign	Internal sign
fire element	one cannot digest food or drink	
aggregate of discrimination	one is no longer mindful of affairs of close persons	
basic wisdom of analysis (our ordinary consciousness mindful of the individual names, purposes and so forth of close persons)	one can no longer remember the names of close persons	appearance of fireflies or sparks within smoke

nose sense	inhalation weak, exhalation strong and lengthy	
odors	one cannot smell	

CHART 4: FOURTH CYCLE OF SIMULTANEOUS DISSOLUTION

Factor dissolving	External sign	Internal sign
wind element	the ten winds move to heart; inhalation and exhalation ceases	
aggregate of compositional factors	one cannot perform physical actions	
basic wisdom of achieving activities (our ordinary consciousness mindful of external activities, purposes and so forth)	one is no longer mindful of external worldly activities, purposes and so forth	appearance of a sputtering butter-lamp about to go out
tongue sense	tongue becomes thick and short; root of tongue becomes blue	
tastes	one cannot experience tastes	
body sense and tangible objects	one cannot experience smoothness or roughness	

CHART 5: FIFTH TO EIGHTH CYCLES OF DISSOLUTION

Factor dissolving	Cause of appearance	Internal sign
FIFTH CYCLE		
eighty conceptions	winds in right and left channels above heart enter central channel at top of head	at first, burning butter-lamp; then, clear vacuity filled with white light
SIXTH CYCLE		
mind of white appearance	winds in right and left channels below heart enter central channel at base of spine	very clear vacuity filled with red light
SEVENTH CYCLE		
mind of red increase	upper and lower winds gather at heart; then winds enter drop at heart	at first, vacuity filled with thick darkness; then as if swooning unconsciously

EIGHTH CYCLE		
mind of black near-attainment	all winds dissolve into the very subtle life-bearing wind in the indestructible drop at the heart	very clear vacuity free of the white, red and black appearances - the mind of clear light of death

Source: Lati Rinbonchay and Jeffrey Hopkins. (1979). Death, Intermediate State and Rebirth in Tibetan Buddhism.

Actual death in the Buddhist tradition, therefore, is "the consciousness permanently leaving the body."[139] Other signs of the consciousness leaving the body are 1) when all heat has left the area of the heart centre (in the centre of the chest), 2) the body starts to smell or decompose, 3) a subtle awareness that the consciousness has left and the body has become like 'an empty shell', 4) a slumping of the body in a practitioner who has been sitting in meditation after the stopping of the breath. Buddhists generally prefer that the body not be removed for disposal before one or more of these signs occur, because until then the consciousness is still in the body and any violent handling of it may disturb the end processes of death. A Buddhist monk or nun or friend should ideally be called in before the body is moved in order for the appropriate prayers and procedures to be carried out.

When the clear light vision ceases, the consciousness leaves the body and passes through the other seven stages of dissolution (black near-attainment, red increase etc.) in reverse order. As soon as this reverse process begins the person is reborn into an intermediate state between lives, with a subtle body that can go instantly wherever it likes, move through solid objects etc., in its journey to the next place of rebirth.

The intermediate state can last from a moment to seven days, depending on whether or not a suitable birthplace is found. If one is not found the being undergoes a "small death," experiencing the eight signs of death as previously described (but very briefly). He/she then again experiences the eight signs of the reverse process and is reborn in a second intermediate state. This can happen for a total of seven births in the intermediate state (making a total of forty-nine days) during which a place of rebirth must be found. The "small death" that occurs between intermediate states or just prior to taking rebirth is compared to experiencing the eight signs (from the mirage-like vision to the clear light), when going into deep sleep or when coming out of a dream. Similarly also, when entering a dream or when awakening from sleep the eight signs of the reverse process are experienced. The Buddhist view is that each living being has a continuity or stream of consciousness that moves from one life to the next. Each being has had countless previous lives and will continue to be reborn again and again without control unless he/she develops his/her mind to the point where, like the yogis mentioned above, he/she gains control over this process. When the stream of consciousness or mind moves from one life to the next it brings with it the karmic imprints or potentialities from previous lives. Karma literally means "action," and all of the actions of body, speech and mind leave an imprint on the mind-stream. These karmas can be negative, positive or neutral, depending on the action. They can ripen at any time in the future, whenever conditions are suitable. These karmic seeds or imprints are never lost.

At the time of death (clear light stage) the consciousness (very subtle mind) leaves the body and the person takes the body of an intermediate state being. They are in the form that they will take in their next life (some texts say the previous life), but in a subtle rather than a gross form. As mentioned previously, it can take up to forty-nine days to find a suitable place of rebirth. This rebirth is propelled by karma and is uncontrolled. In effect the karma of the intermediate state being matches that of its future parents. The intermediate state being has the illusory appearance of its future parents copulating. It is drawn to this place by the force of attraction to its parent of the opposite sex, and it is this desire that causes the consciousness of the intermediate state being to enter the fertilized ovum. This happens at or near the time of conception and the new life has begun.

To encapsulate, here are the key points to remember:

❖ The teaching of Buddha holds that all of us will pass away eventually as part of the natural process of birth.

- ◆ To Buddhists, death is not the end of life; it is merely the end of the body we inhabit in this life. Our spirit will still remain and seek out the attachment to a new body and a new life.

- ◆ Buddhism is a belief that emphasizes the impermanence of life, including those beyond the present life. With this in mind Buddhists do not fear death as it will lead to rebirth.

- ◆ Consideration for the dying will vary depending on the Buddhist Group

- ◆ Most important consideration relates to the state of mind at the time of death. This will influence how the individual will experience rebirth.

Spiritual Care of the Dying

- ◆ If patient has specific religious beliefs, these can be utilized to help them.

- ◆ If patient does not have specific religious beliefs, he or she can be encouraged to have positive or virtuous thoughts at the time of death, such as reminding him or her of positive things s/he has done during his or her life.

- ◆ For a spiritual practitioner, it is helpful to encourage him or her to have thoughts such as love, compassion, remembering their spiritual teacher.

- ◆ It is beneficial to have an image in the room of Jesus, Mary, Buddha, or some other spiritual figure that may have meaning for the dying person.

- ◆ It may be helpful for those caring for the dying person to say some prayers, recite mantras, etc.

- ◆ Before and at the moment of death, the monk, nun or spiritual friends will read prayers and chants from Buddhist Scriptures.

- ◆ One needs to be sensitive to the needs of the dying person. The most important thing, according to the tradition, is to keep the mind of the person happy and calm. Nothing should be done (including certain spiritual practices) if this causes the person to be annoyed or irritated.

- ❖ There is a common conception that it is good to read "The Tibetan Book of the Dead" to the dying person, but if s/he is not familiar with the particular deities and practices contained in it, then this is not likely to prove very beneficial.

- ❖ Because the death process is so important, it is best not to disturb the dying person with noise or shows of emotion. Expressing attachment and clinging to the dying person can disturb the mind and therefore the death process, so it is more helpful to mentally let the person go, to encourage them to move on to the next life without fear. It is important not to deny death or to push it away, just to be with the dying person as fully and openly as possible, trying to have an open and deep sharing of the person's fear, pain, joy, love, etc.

When Death Has Occurred

- ❖ When death is imminent the family may call in the Buddhist priest to pray so that at the final moment, the right state of mind has been generated and the person can find their way into a higher state of rebirth as they leave the present life.

- ❖ The nurses and family members should not touch the body – wait three to eight hours after breathing ceases before touching the body for any preparation after death.

- ❖ Buddhists believe that the spirit of the persons will linger on for some time and can be affected by what happens to the body.

- ❖ It is very pertinent to mention that neither the nurse nor the physician needs to worry about how to respond to the spiritual or religious requests of the patient or family members. It is assumed, I hope, that most hospitals have the department so designated as pastoral or spiritual care to cater to such an important aspect of the human person. Hence, the hospital chaplains would serve as great resources either in providing such services or in contacting outside clergy to meet the needs of the dying patient and the comfort of the family.

Death & Dying in Hinduism

Hinduism: Brief Insight

"Hindu suffering can be perplexing to Western thought. With almost 2.3 million Hindus of Indian origin and an additional 1 million practicing American Hindus now in the United States, healthcare practitioners need to know more about the tenets of Hinduism to provide culturally sensitive care. Family and community interconnectedness, karma, and reincarnation are major beliefs of Hinduism. Healthcare decisions may be made by the most senior family member or the eldest son. Karma is a combination of cosmic and moral cause and effect that can cross lifetimes and life lessons learned for spiritual growth. The belief in reincarnation gives great comfort to the dying and their families because they believe their loved ones will be reborn into a new life and that they are not gone forever. Enduring physical suffering may lead to spiritual growth and a more fortunate rebirth."[140] It is important to mention that Hinduism is the oldest known religion, having been practiced over 8000 years.[141] As it may be included in the religious demographics of many hospitals or caregiving communities, it is poignant to note that several newer religions have roots in Hinduism such as Jainism (around 3000 BCE); Buddhism (around 600 BCE); Sikhism (around 16th century); and Brahmoism (around 18th century).[142] According to historians, Hinduism has no founder, no beginning that can be pointed to, and no one holy book. The most holy Hindu text, Subramuniyaswami writes, is called the Veda: a word that means wisdom. Other holy texts are called the Upanishads and the Puranas.[143] According to Jeste and Vahia, the Bhagavad-Gita (song of God) is the most recent of the sacred texts and the most practical, giving devotees a more practical guide to Vedic wisdom.[144]

Highlights of Hinduism

- ❖ Oldest known religion still in practice
- ❖ Belief in one God with many forms
- ❖ Spirituality is a way of life for Hindus
- ❖ Family is very important, and healthcare decisions are often made communally with the senior family member or eldest son as the final authority
- ❖ Karma is moral cause and effect of thoughts and actions
- ❖ Reincarnation means being born into a new existence on earth to evolve spiritually
- ❖ Adherence to traditional values depends largely on acculturation.[145]

Spiritual Suffering

"Suffering for the Hindu is highly related to the concept of karma."[146] As Subramuniyaswami pointed out, "Belief in karma and reincarnation are strong forces at work in the Hindu mind." That is, any good or bad thought or action leads to reward or punishment either in this life or a future existence, Thrane states.

Spiritual suffering for a Hindu, according to Susan Thrane, comes from knowing at the end of life that responsibilities are left undone, karmic tasks are not completed, or bad thoughts and deeds predominated. The concept of karma conveys that suffering is part of life. Suffering is a result of past thoughts and actions either in this life or a previous life. By enduring suffering, a Hindu "pays for" or cancels past negative actions. "Suffering can be positive if it leads to progress on a spiritual path, to be tested and learn from a difficult experience."[147] Susan Thrane opines correctly that what may appear to be needless suffering to Western minds, especially clinicians, may be in fact, a striving to meet death in a clear and conscious state and may be an attempt to atone for karmic debt. Hence, there is the need for greater understanding from care providers in view of the religious perspective of the Hindu-patient or "delayed" decision making by family members. Based on Hindu belief, Hindus who feel they need to diminish or alleviate past karma may wish to endure suffering. This may involve fasting, doing penance such as intense prayer or worship, or enduring pain even when medication is available.[148] As part of holistic care, it is essential, as Thrane pointed out, that care providers assist patient and family to be able to complete their religious ceremonies, prayer, or penance as these may be very important to their spiritual wellbeing. Also, she suggests further, assisting the patient and family does not necessarily mean participating; it can simply mean helping them to find the materials, assuring them that they will not be disturbed, or making a timely and appropriate referrals. Respecting, allowing private time and space for these religious activities will be helpful, states Thrane.

Death & Dying Practices

Death is the fulfillment of this life and a chance for a better reincarnation, a chance to learn new karmic lessons and to move closer to moksha (becoming one with Brahman – God). Hindus believe that death must come naturally at the proper time. Life should not be prolonged by aggressive medical means unless it will result in a good quality of life. Prolonging life artificially would result in the soul remaining on earth past its natural time "tethered to a lower astral region rather than being released into higher astral/mental levels."[149] Hindus will often forgo aggressive treatment when an illness is terminal or there is no hope of recovery. If the patient is a parent of young children, more aggressive treatments are often sought in the hope of prolonging life to provide for the children. Nor should life be cut short willfully. Speeding up death by artificial means would result in a large karmic debt. Suicide would result in many lesser rebirths to "make up" for the karmic debt of ending one's life unnaturally.[150]

As it is customary to the faith, Hindus may endure pain or uncomfortable symptoms to face death with a clear mind. [151] Ideally, a

Hindu should die at home surrounded by family and friends who will sing sacred hymns and say prayers or chant the dying person's mantra in his/her right ear if he/she is unconscious. As death approaches, the bed should be turned so the head faces east. Hindus with a terminal illness or certain other disabling conditions are allowed to choose a "self-willed death by fasting."[152] This is an acceptable method of ending suffering, Susan Thrane surmises.

Final Hints to Remember:

- ❖ In view of End-of-Life (EOL): Hindus are very family oriented; and so, may have many visitors at one time. There may be singing, chanting, praying, reading from holy books, and sharing food.
- ❖ For Power-of-Attorney (POA): Healthcare decisions will likely be made by a senior family member or eldest son.
- ❖ Palliative and hospice care are aligned with Hindu values.
- ❖ Hindus believe that death should neither be sought nor prolonged.
- ❖ Spiritual suffering is connected to karma. Enduring physical suffering at the end-of-life may reverse bad karma.
- ❖ Hindus would like to die at home surrounded by family. Ideally, they would like to be conscious and be thinking of Brahman at the very moment of death.
- ❖ If the person is unconscious, it would be helpful to have the eldest son or a senior family member chanting the person's mantra (sacred phrase) in his/her right ear prior to death.[153]

DEATH & DYING IN CHRISTIAN TRADITION

Different Christian Groups Represented: In discussing the issue of death and dying in a Christian tradition, it is important to state from the outset that it might be practically impossible to have a comprehensive list of all Christian denominations all over the globe. That would be an overwhelming task to accomplish. Hence, without much ado, the list of various Christian denominations below is by no means exhaustive. Additionally, the list follows alphabetical chronology and is not, in any way, an order of superiority – if there is any such thing.

- African Methodist Episcopal
- African Methodist Episcopal Zion
- Amish
- Assembly of God
- Baptist
- Brethren
- Catholicism
- Christian Church (The Disciples of Christ)
- Christian Methodist Episcopal
- Christian Science
- Church of Christ (Independent)
- Episcopal Greek Orthodox
- Independent Conservative Evangelical
- Lutheran
- Mennonite
- Moravian
- Mormon (Church of Jesus Christ of Latter-Day Saints)
- Pentecostal
- Presbyterian
- Seventh Day Adventist
- Society of Friends (Quakers)
- Unitarian Universalist
- United Church of Christ
- United Methodist

Helping the Dying to Prepare: What to Expect, What to do

First and foremost, Christians, like many other religions, understand that dying is a process. The process often involves fears and loneliness, not necessarily fear of death but the fear of the "unknown destination" or "after-life here on earth." As shared earlier, a patient once shared her fears with me: "I'm afraid of what's after this life!" I was invited to visit the patient by her longtime friends because, as they said, "She's afraid of dying." The patient, God rest her in peace, did affirm her fear but not of death itself or dying but the fate after death has occurred.

That being said, however, there might be a possibility of thanatophobia, that is, the fear of death. Another patient stated, "I'm afraid of nightfall." His wife had requested that a chaplain stop by every night to have moments of prayer with him due to his expressed fear and inability to sleep at nights. During my spiritual care conversation with him, he shared with me that he "cannot sleep at night for the fear that I might not wake again…I'm afraid that I will die." It was so helpful, as confirmed by both patient and wife, that on-call chaplains could spend some moments of prayer with him as requested, dousing his fear and bringing calmness and hopefulness. Similar situations as these two stories stand as a clear indication that the patient needs some spiritual assistance and that caregivers need to help. In order to aid in the peaceful dying process effectively, care providers and caregivers might need to know and understand the following fundamentals:

- The dying process affects the psychosocial roles and attitudes of the people involved. That is, from a religious standpoint, there may be positive or negative impacts by family members, on the dying. For instance, individual or family's concept of "salvation." It is not unusual that a patient might be subjected to religious "judgment" within the religious framework of "self-righteousness." Some patients have been subjected to receiving, not so much what they'd love to receive spiritually perhaps, but the fulfillment of the family's desire or religious wish for them. For instance, an eighty-four-year man received baptism upon the request of his wife while in Intensive Care Unit (ICU). Did he long to be baptized? It's debatable! It is important to inquire from the patient, if alert and oriented, how the journey is affecting him or her and what could be done to help ensure peaceful transition. When a patient is at the "mercy" of his/her family or POA (Power of Attorney), care providers can only go by their requests and/or rejections.

- Is the person "ready" to die or not? Some dying patients can be very selfless – life and death isn't so much about them, but their primary concern is how it might impact their loved ones, those to be left behind. Hence, some patients simply need to be assured that their family will be okay. Even when sedated and visibly unconscious, dying patients who have cultivated such a morale and caring attitude all through their lives would need to hear the words of assurance and reassurance repeatedly from their loved ones. Some people want to make sure that their spouse is going to be able to function once they die. Some people need assurance that their lives have had meaning and that when they die they are going to be "okay" – not going to "hell" or into nothingness. Some need assurance that God will be there waiting for them. Care providers/families can help hold the **"Assurance Bridge"** in preparation for less fearful crossover. Gestures such as physical touching; comforting words ("it's okay;" "we'll be okay;" "don't be afraid" etc); delightful/favorite songs; family-bond/unity reinforced or assured, etc. might be helpful.

- **Mortality:** For most Christians, dying might be interpreted as a "necessary bridge" to transit into eternal life. That is, both the concept and the theology of 'death' are not strange in the religious understanding of Christian tradition. As a matter of fact, the theology of eternal life is predicated on the necessity or the inevitability of death – the cessation of breath (life). An overriding concern for the dying and family is a "good" death. What is a "good" death? The Institute of Medicine defined a good death as "one that is free from avoidable suffering for patients, families and caregivers in general in accordance with the patients' and families' wishes."[154]

Based on studies, here are some top concerns:

- Pain and symptom management (rated #1 on almost every study)
- Clear decision making
- Avoiding inappropriate prolongation of dying but without physician-assisted or euthanasia or "mercy killing."
- Preparation for death: putting one's house in order.
- Relieving burdens
- Strengthening relationships with loved ones, including reconciliation and forgiveness.
- A sense of completion: some people rate their existence and life as "successful" based on their ability to complete their life aspirations and accomplishments. Hence, it is not unusual to

encounter patients who would consider that they've failed or display some negative feelings about themselves due to their low sense of completion. Validation of even little efforts might be of great help here.

- ❖ Contributing to others
- ❖ An affirmation as a whole person
- ❖ Assurance of funeral arrangements
- ❖ Being mentally aware
- ❖ At peace with God

A Gallup poll in May, 1997, found the following major spiritual concerns of Americans about death:

- ❖ Concern and % positive responses
- ❖ Not being forgiven by God – 56%
- ❖ Not being reconciled with others – 56%
- ❖ Dying while being cut off or removed from God or a higher power – 51%
- ❖ Not being forgiven by someone for a past offense – 49%
- ❖ Not having a blessing from a family member or clergy – 39%
- ❖ The nature of the experience of death – 39%
- ❖ With these, a "good" death may vary.
- ❖ What to do? Kindly ask what he/she/they think a good death is, then help facilitate what they consider as important to have a good death.

"Decision Time" vs. Hope for Miracle

Undoubtedly, hospitalization can lead to the experience of crises for patients as well as family members. The crises can certainly take multidimensional turns – physical, psychological, emotional, and spiritual. Patient and families seek "quick" fixes and speedy return to a normal course of life. This is much more likely when the hospitalization incident happens suddenly, leaving no one to prepare and put all affairs in proper order. So many courses of daily events are suspended and regimens altered. In addition to this fast-moving course of events is the expectation from the hospital community – the primary care providers – for family members to "step up" and assume great responsibility for which they never prepared, or at least did not expect at this point in time. Some can easily freak out and experience mental freeze. Incontestably, time is of the essence in medical urgency. However, when the pressure is on, there is an unimaginable magnitude of anxiety, worry and confusion, to say the least. Experience has shown that some family members are "boxed" into panic attack and a possible loss of control. When the failure of the human body springs its surprise, it is relatively difficult both for the "victim" and family members to keep balance amidst several hospital demands – signing of consent forms, providing documents such as "Advance Directives" or "Final Wishes", appointing POA (Power of Attorney); stepping up to assuming decision-making roles, etc. This "strange" role can be demanding, especially when the patient remains intubated and unconscious in the Intensive Care Unit (ICU). It is more difficult, for instance on the spouse, when the patient has no advance directives and a critical health situation has continually eluded their spousal conversations. This was the case at a family meeting of an 89-year-old patient whose wife said that they had never discussed such end-of-life (EOL) issues. It was hard on the family – wife, children and in-laws – to arrive at a decision, within the tenets of being the patient's voice and advocate.

For patients who have prepared their advance directives or final wishes, as some hospitals call it, decision making at critical points of illness are "easier" on family members, especially when they are physically silent or unable to verbalize their wishes due to the nature of the prevailing condition. A family could be caught between knowing/doing the "right thing" and not wanting to be "responsible" for their loved one's death. These are the unspoken struggles family members face in ICU or other EOL situations amidst the call from attending physician to make a decision. It is partly, also, the reason the POA or other family member so involved might "desperately" wish for a miracle to happen. For such a conflicted caregiver, issues for decision are pushed off or postponed; there may be a perceivable communication gap between the family and the physician.

Amidst these matters, therefore, the dying and his/her family could sometimes feel "pressured" by their care providers: "Decision time." It is not unusual for Christians to hope for "miracles" even in the face of obvious imminent death. Faith is usually invoked; Biblical references are often remembered and quoted; and a family spiritual leader often consulted. This is consistent with Christian faith tradition – human expectation of Divine intervention amidst odds, storms and crises of life. Care providers should exercise patience, compassion, understanding, and help to limit anxieties surrounding imminent death. Do miracles happen in hospitals? Yes! Do they happen all the time? No! Patients and families understand that. But who knows whose turn it may be to narrate the "miracle story!" This is strictly in the domain of spiritual purview; hence, a call for spiritual care consults for appropriate intervention.

The Final Journey: Responding to the Spiritual Needs of the Dying

- **Spiritual Bridge:** Caring pastor or chaplain is a symbol of religious faith and an active spiritual life.
- His or her presence and tangible ministry are much appreciated and welcomed.
- The pastor represents assurance, comfort, and hope in a time of great uncertainty, transition, and need.
- Amidst fears and loneliness, the dying looks to the spiritual figure: help in communicating with his or her family, guidance

in reflecting on the quality of life, comfort in a major transition.

- ❖ Survivors look to their pastor for help with family arrangements, funeral and burial planning.

Christians' Rites & Rituals

- ❖ It is appropriate to ask patients if they have any rituals that are especially important to them and if they wish to observe those rituals.

- ❖ It is also appropriate to ask family members if they have any family rituals that they would like to observe with their loved one who is dying.

- ❖ It is very important, however, that you do not impose a ritual, not even prayer, on a patient or family that does not want it. It is not about the care provider; rather, it is about the patient and/or family. Religious zeal needs to be curtailed.

- ❖ If you're not sure of a patient's or family's religious affiliation, kindly ask.

- ❖ Even if you know, try not to assume that because the patient is "Catholic," for example, that he or she would want a priest, or would need the Last Rite. Or because they are of different culture or ethnicity that they will want something that I can or cannot offer them. We let them teach us what they do and how they do it.

- ❖ Suffice it to say that "family is the expert on how they cope and how they grieve." Observation may be a useful tool in this process.

Sacrament of the Sick and/or Last Rites is very important in the Catholic faith tradition. If a patient is a Roman Catholic and expresses the desire to receive the Last Rite or his/her family does, a priest should be contacted forthwith. The priest discerns, upon the situation at hand, what is appropriate to administer – Sacrament of the Sick and/or Last Rites. It may be offensive for a Catholic or the family to be denied the ritual of Sacrament of the Sick (SS) or Last Rites (for the dying), and it may place heavy "guilt" on the family if delayed or denied. This is not the same as "praying with the patient or family" as some clinicians or even chaplains might intend. Some other Christian denominations also have various forms of anointing. It may be appropriate to call the chaplain or the patient's pastor in such a situation.

For Christian Science: There are no physical rituals or sacraments in Christian Science. A member may want to be in touch with a Christian Science practitioner.[155]

For other Christians: Kindly respond to their request for a chaplain/pastor for spiritual support/prayers/Rites/Rituals for their dying loved one and/or for family at this difficult moment. In general, the presence of family and friends brings comfort during the dying process. Telling the story of the deceased brings release and insight into the joy and sorrow of the parting. Christian mourners turn to worship, experience the comfort of scripture, and offer sacraments for healing.

Rites & Rituals: Emergency Baptism

The desired goal of this book wouldn't be achieved without devoting a brief section to emergency baptism in the hospital. Baptism, a common religious rite shared by most Christian denominations and groups, can pose a great challenge to religiously inclined healthcare workers especially during EOL situations on Neonatal Intensive Care Unit (NICU) for infants. It is not unusual for some nurses, respiratory therapists, or other clinicians to be so concerned for the "salvation" of the patient (the baby) that they desire that he or she be baptized. Since some clinicians are also religious leaders in their respective churches or communities, they sometimes collapse the professional walls and boundaries by pushing forward to baptize dying babies, even without the request of the baby's parent or family or guardian. This, according to history, has brought lawsuit against some hospitals in the States.

It must be said, unequivocally, that hospitals are extraordinary places for conferring sacraments upon the believers, including Baptism. Churches are ordinary places for sacramental celebrations. By extraordinary, it means that priests and ministers are granted the "faculty" or ministerial authority to perform such holy rites when death is imminent, that is, life is in danger. In such a dire spiritual and religious need, anyone can perform such a rite, as appropriate, doing so with the mind of the recipient's faith community. In the event that death is imminent, note the following before you proceed to administer emergent baptism for babies and un-baptized adults:

- **Infant Baptism** is a crucial belief to Roman Catholics. However, offer the parent(s) the opportunity to decide for/against baptizing the baby upon delivery. A priest should be contacted immediately to be on standby, or chaplain on-call should be contacted for the same purpose. In the event that neither a priest nor a chaplain is available or can be reached, anyone can perform the rites of baptism (on emergency), including the parent, or the nurse, etc.

- **Un-Baptized Adult:** This should be encouraged only in extreme cases, that is, when death is imminent upon the patient and patient's family has so requested. The same procedure, as stated above, holds.

- **Do not baptize** a baby without express permission from parent(s)/guardian/! The rule of thumb: Remember that it is not what you (the clinician) want, but what the child's parent or caregiver wants.

- **The Rites:** In the event of emergency baptism, pour ordinary water on the forehead of the one to be baptized three times while you say the following words: "I baptize you in the Name of the Father, and of the Son, and of the Holy Spirit."

- Lastly, a word about the staff of the hospital:

- Care-providers, such as physicians, nurses, tech, etc, have spent a lot of time caring for the patient and family. So it is not unusual to be present in the room for last rituals, rites or prayers. It gives the staff an opportunity for some closure, enables the family to thank the staff, and for the staff to express their condolences to the family.[156]

When Death Occurs

For some individuals, death is the worst aspect of life. However, people's view of death is shaped by their cultural background, religious beliefs, community heritage, social norms, personal philosophy, and individual worldview: some view death as a real stranger or an aggressive intruder into normal living while some view it, including pain and suffering, as integral parts of life. The latter group might be able to reconcile the concept of dying with the idea of living. To them, "death virtually gives meaning to life."

Hence, when death occurs, different reactions abound: wailing and rolling, sobbing, non-visible tears, "emotionless or indifference," etc. Only the individual knows and is able to explain the depth of the loss and the chosen way(s) to express such. Since a bereaved person might have a delayed reaction to his/her loss, it will be helpful, for care providers, to be mindful of this and kindly respect the emotional feelings and loss the deceased family members might be passing through. It is pertinent to mention this since, as I have witnessed, some clinicians and care providers have expressed "surprise" at the minimal physical display by a wife who had just lost her husband. Shedding tears or physical emotional display is perhaps one of several ways of showing a great loss!

Christian *Rites* may be appropriate for the deceased, as family requests. For instance, a Roman Catholic may request the Last Rites or the Final Commendation – Prayer for the Dead. Other Christians may request the presence of their pastors or a hospital chaplain for the purpose of prayer or any Rites that they may deem appropriate. Suffice it to say that Christians, in general, would prefer to be offered the opportunity to receive a comforting presence of a religious or spiritual leader who could minister to their spiritual needs, as they grieve their loss and also be assured of God's mercy and forgiveness for the dead, in the hope of resurrection.

Here's the ***Key***: If and only if it is okay for the family or the bereaved to have a chaplain called. Some families, as I have seen, have expressed surprise and dismay when a chaplain shows up in the patient's room without the family's prior knowledge or request. That the patient was religious does not automatically mean that family would follow suit. Often, the deceased, like an unconscious patient, is left at the "mercy" of the survived families.

The ***Goal***: to support the bereaved as they express grief and loss in their own MOST COMFORTABLE WAY.

Death and Dying in Islamic Tradition

Faith Foundation about death: "Allah is the One who gives life and takes it away, at a time appointed by Him."

Islamic Tradition and the Dying:

When a person is dying, relatives and close friends are normally present. Because Islam recognizes no intermediaries between humans and God, it has, strictly speaking, no clergy. Not even the Sufis, who claimed to look after the spiritual life of their followers…could claim to mediate on behalf of the dying by administering sacraments.[157] ***Obligations from friends and relatives:*** the dying person will expect to be visited by friends and relatives, who are encouraged to pray for his or her welfare in the life to come. Islamic tradition encourages a large number of visitors. Hence, strict adherence to "two visitors per bed" will cause difficulty for all concerned. Members of the immediate family will often stay by the bedside reciting from the Qur'an. Thus, availability of the Qur'an would be considered a kind gesture.[158]

Repentance on deathbed is unacceptable in Islam. The dying person recites the confession of the faith. "There is no god but God and Muhammad is his messenger." If he or she has done some wrong to anyone, the forgiveness of that person is sought, if possible, for according to Islamic doctrine, "Fulfilling the rights of people has priority over the rights of God, and God will not forgive violation of human rights unless those wronged have forgiven."[159]

When a Muslim is near death, those around him or her are called upon to give comfort, and reminders of God's mercy and forgiveness. They may recite verses from the Qur'an, give physical comfort, and encourage the dying one to recite words of remembrance and prayer. It is recommended, if possible, for a Muslim's last words to be the declaration of faith: "I bear witness that there is no god but Allah."[160]

Islam and Mortality:

"For a Muslim, death marks the transition from one state of existence to the next. Islam teaches that life on earth is an examination – the life to come is the eternal abode where one will reap the fruit of one's endeavors on earth. Death is therefore not to be resisted or fought against, but rather something to be accepted as part of the overall divine plan. Deliberate euthanasia is prohibited. However, it is pertinent to note that "undue suffering has no place in Islam and if death is hastened in the process of giving adequate analgesia then this is allowed." What is important is that the primary intent is not to hasten death."[161]

In counseling of Muslims regarding a terminal illness, or relatives after bereavement, these points should be borne in mind:

- ❖ Death according to the Qur'an, is a mere link or a passage between two segments of a continuous life: "God receives the souls when they die and those who do not die he receives them in their sleep; he then keeps those for whom he has decreed death while others he releases until the appointed term…" (39, 42).

- ❖ When death has occurred, the Prophet's traditions enjoin burial of the dead without unnecessary delay, burial rights being simple and austere. Wailing loudly for the dead is forbidden.

- Islamic doctrine strictly forbids wailing for the dead or observance of their death beyond three days in most Muslim societies pre-Islamic customs still prevail (elaborate ceremonies).

- That is, it is forbidden for those in mourning to excessively wail, scream, or thrash about. However, grief is normal when one has lost a loved one, and it is natural and weeping is permitted.

- A ceremony is observed universally in Muslim countries on the third and often also on the 40th day after the death of a dear one; the Qur'an-recitation *in completo* is done, and guests who participate in the recitations are given food.[162]

In brief:

- "For a Muslim, death marks the transition from one state of existence to the next. Islam teaches that life on earth is an examination – the life to come is the eternal abode where one will reap the fruit of one's endeavors on earth.

- Death is therefore not to be resisted or fought against, but rather something to be accepted as part of the overall divine plan. Deliberate euthanasia is prohibited. However, it is pertinent to note that "undue suffering has no place in Islam and if death is hastened in the process of giving adequate analgesia then this is allowed." What is important is that the primary intent is not to hasten death."

What to do when a Muslim is dying?

As said earlier on, Islam recognizes no intermediaries between humans and Allah. Hence, care providers should note the following within the tenets of the Islamic tradition:

- No clergy that mediates on behalf of the dying. However, the dying or his or her family could request an Imam. This religious/spiritual request does not contradict the initial stated position of the religion in view of an intermediary between Allah and humans. It further confirms in some variations that it is permissible according to the practice of the faith and the individual's spiritual tendencies.

- ❖ The dying person recites the confession of the faith: "There is no god but Allah and Muhammad is his messenger."

- ❖ When a Muslim is near death, those around him or her are called upon to give comfort, and reminders of God's mercy and forgiveness.

- ❖ They may recite verses from the Qur'an, give physical comfort, and encourage the dying one to recite words of remembrance and prayer.

- ❖ It is recommended, if possible, for a Muslim's last words to be the declaration of faith: "I bear witness that there is no god but Allah."

- ❖ *Kalima-e-Shahadah* (Creed of Islam)

- ❖ For a dying Muslim, it is customary that the recitation of "the declaration of faith" is offered. Also, the dying patient should be turned on his/her right side.[163]

When Death Occurs:

- ❖ Simply say: "From Allah we come, to Allah we'll return." Close the eyes, prepare to wash the body (*Ghusl*), and say good things about the deceased.[164]

- ❖ In preparation for burial, the family or care provider will wash and shroud the body. However, if the deceased was killed (as a martyr), this step is not performed; he/she is buried in the clothes they died in

- ❖ The deceased will be washed respectfully, with clean and scented water, in a manner similar to how Muslims make ablutions for prayer. The body will then be wrapped in sheets of clean, white cloth (the *kafan*)

- ❖ Post mortem is not allowed in Islam as this would prolong the stay of the body after death and delay the prescribed time for burial.

- When death has occurred, the Prophet's traditions enjoin burial of the dead without unnecessary delay, burial rights being simple and austere. Wailing loudly for the dead is forbidden.

RELIGIOUS VIEWS ON ORGAN, TISSUE AND BLOOD DONATION[165]

Charity + Love + Compassion = Neighbor-*in*-Need

All major religions in the U.S. support the principles of donation and transplantation. In each religion, however, there are different schools of thought, which mean views may differ (donatelifeen.org). Suffice it to say that although the vast majority of religious' views will be presented in this book; however, this does not represent the entirety of religions throughout the world. Also, the author concurs with the alphabetical listing of religions by donate-life organizations on its webpage, rather than being considered in order of importance.

AME & AME Zion (African Methodist Episcopal)

Organ and tissue donation is viewed as an act of neighborly love and charity by these denominations. They encourage all members to support donation as a way of helping others.

AMISH

The Amish will consent to transplantation if they believe it is for the well-being of the transplant recipient. John Hostetler, world renowned authority on Amish religion and professor of anthropology at Temple University in Philadelphia, says in his book, Amish Society, "The Amish believe that since God created the human body, it is God who heals." However, nothing in the Amish understanding of the Bible forbids them from using modern medical services, including surgery, hospitalization, dental work, anesthesia, blood transfusions or immunization.

ASSEMBLY OF GOD

The Church has no official policy regarding organ and tissue donation. The decision to donate is left up to the individual. Donation is highly supported by the denomination.

BAHA'I

The Baha'i regards organ donation as praiseworthy: the wishes of the patient and next of kin should be ascertained, and consent obtained.

BAPTIST

Though Baptists generally believe that organ and tissue donation and transplantation are ultimately matters of personal conscience, the nation's largest protestant denomination, the Southern Baptist Convention, adopted a resolution in 1988 encouraging physicians to request organ donation in appropriate circumstances and to "…encourage voluntarism regarding organ donations in the spirit of stewardship, compassion for the needs of others and alleviating suffering." Other Baptist groups have supported organ and tissue donation as an act of charity and leave the decision to donate up to the individual.

BRETHREN

While no official position has been taken by the Brethren denominations, according to Pastor Mike Smith, there is a consensus among the National Fellowship of Grace Brethren that organ and tissue donation is a charitable act so long as it does not impede the life or hasten the death of the donor or does not come from an unborn child.

BUDDHISM

Buddhists believe that organ and tissue donation is a matter of individual conscience and place high value on acts of compassion. Reverend Gyomay

Massao, president and founder of the Buddhist Temple of Chicago, says, "We honor those people who donate their bodies and organs to the advancement of medical science and to saving lives."

CATHOLICISM

Roman Catholics view organ and tissue donation as an act of charity and love. Transplants are morally and ethically acceptable to the Vatican. Pope Benedict XVI proclaimed: "To be an organ donor means to carry out an act of love toward someone in need, toward a brother in difficulty. It is a free act of love that every person of good will can do at any time and for any brother."

CHRISTIAN CHURCH (Disciples of Christ)

The Christian Church encourages organ and tissue donation, stating that we were created for God's glory and for sharing God's love. A 1985 resolution, adopted by the General Assembly, encourages "…members of the Christian Church (Disciples of Christ) to enroll as organ donors and prayerfully support those who have received an organ transplant."

CHRISTIAN SCIENCE

The Church of Christ Scientist does not have a specific position regarding organ donation. According to the First Church of Christ Scientist in Boston, Christian Scientists normally rely on spiritual instead of medical means of healing. They are free, however, to choose whatever form of medical treatment they desire – including a transplant. The question of organ and tissue donation is an individual decision.

CHURCH OF CHRIST (Independent)

Generally, they have no opposition to organ and tissue donation. Each church is autonomous and leaves the decision to donate up to the individual.

EPISCOPAL

The Episcopal Church passed a resolution in 1982 that recognizes the life-giving benefits of organ, blood and tissue donation. All Christians are encouraged to become organ, blood and tissue donors "…as part of their ministry to others in the name of Christ, who gave His life that we may have life in its fullness."

GREEK ORTHODOX

According to Reverend Dr. Milton Efthimiou, Director of the Department of Church and Society for the Greek Orthodox Church of North and South America, "The Greek Orthodox Church is not opposed to organ donation as long as the organs and tissue in questions are used to better human life, i.e., for transplantation or for research that will lead to improvements in the treatment and prevention of disease."

GYPSIES

Gypsies are a people of different ethnic groups without a formalized religion. They share common folk beliefs and tend to be opposed to organ donation. Their opposition is connected with their beliefs about the afterlife. Traditional belief contends that for one year after death the soul retraces its steps. Thus, the body must remain intact because the soul maintains its physical shape.

HINDUISM

According to the Hindu Temple Society of North America, Hindus are not prohibited by religious law from donating their organs. This act is an individual's decision. H.L. Trivedi, in Transplantation Proceedings, stated that, "Hindu mythology has stories in which the parts of the human body are used for the benefit of other humans and society. There is nothing in the Hindu religion indicating that parts of humans, dead or alive, cannot be used to alleviate the suffering of other humans."

INDEPENDENT CONSERVATIVE EVANGELICAL

Generally, Evangelicals have no opposition to organ and tissue donation. Each church is autonomous and leaves the decision to donate up to the individual.

ISLAM

Islam as a religion believes in the principle of saving human lives. According to A. Sachedina in his Transplantation Proceedings (1990) article, Islamic Views on Organ Transplantation, "...the majority of the Muslim scholars belonging to various schools of Islamic law have invoked the principle of priority of saving human life and have permitted the organ transplant as a necessity to procure that noble end."

JEHOVAH'S WITNESSES

According to the Watch Tower Society, Jehovah's Witnesses believe donation is a matter of individual decision. Jehovah's Witnesses are often assumed to be opposed to donation because of their belief against blood transfusion. However, this merely means that all blood must be removed from the organs and tissues before being transplanted.

JUDAISM

All four branches of Judaism (Orthodox, Conservative, Reform and Reconstructionist) support and encourage donation. According to Orthodox Rabbi Moses Tendler, Chairman of the Biology Department of Yeshiva University in New York City and Chairman of the Bioethics Commission of the Rabbinical Council of America, "If one is in the position to donate an organ to save another's life, it's obligatory to do so, even if the donor never knows who the beneficiary will be. The basic principle of Jewish ethics – 'the infinite worth of the human being'- also includes donation of corneas, since eyesight restoration is considered a life-saving operation." In 1991, the Rabbinical Council of America

(Orthodox) approved organ donations as permissible, and even required, from brain-dead patients. The Reform movement looks upon the transplant program favorably and Rabbi Richard Address, Director of the Union of American Hebrew Congregations Bio-Ethics Committee and Committee on Older Adults, states: "Judaic Response materials provide a positive approach and by and large the North American Reform Jewish community approves of transplantation."

LUTHERAN

In 1984, the Lutheran Church in America passed a resolution stating that donation contributes to the well-being of humanity and can be "...an expression of sacrificial love for a neighbor in need." They call on members to consider donating organs and to make any necessary family and legal arrangements, including the use of a signed donor card.

MENNONITE

Mennonites have no formal position on donation, but are not opposed to it. They believe the decision to donate is up to the individual and/or his or her family.

MORAVIAN

The Moravian Church has made no statement addressing organ and tissue donation or transplantation. Robert E. Sawyer, President, Provincial Elders Conference, Moravian Church of America, Southern Province, states: "There is nothing in our doctrine or policy that would prevent a Moravian pastor from assisting a family in making a decision to donate or not to donate an organ." It is, therefore, a matter of individual choice.

MORMON (Church of Jesus Christ of Latter-day Saints)

The Church of Jesus Christ of Latter-day Saints statement: "The donation of organs and tissue is a selfless act that often results in great benefit to individuals with medical conditions. The decision to will or donate one's own body organs or tissue for medical purposes, or the decision to authorize the transplant of organs or tissue from a deceased family member, is made by the individual or the deceased member's family. The decision to receive a donated organ should be made after receiving competent medical counsel and confirmation through prayer."

PENTECOSTAL

Pentecostals believe that the decision to donate be left up to the individual.

PRESBYTERIAN

Presbyterians encourage and support donation. They respect a person's right to make decisions regarding his or her own body.

SEVENTH-DAY ADVENTIST

Donation and transplantation are strongly encouraged by Seventh-Day Adventists. They have many transplant hospitals, including Loma Linda in California. Loma Linda specializes in pediatric heart transplantation.

SHINTO

In Shinto, the dead body is considered to be impure and dangerous, and thus quite powerful. "In folk belief context, injuring a dead body is a serious crime…" according to E. Namihira in his article, Shinto Concept Concerning the Dead Human Body. "To this day it is difficult to obtain consent from bereaved families for organ donation or dissection for medical education or pathological anatomy…the Japanese regard them all in the sense of injuring a dead body." Families are often concerned that they not injure the itai, the relationship between the dead person and the bereaved people.

SIKH

The Sikh religion stresses the importance of performing noble deeds, and saving a life is considered one of the greatest forms of noble deeds. Therefore, organ donation is deemed acceptable to the Sikh religion.

SOCIETY OF FRIENDS (Quakers)

Organ and tissue donation is believed to be an individual decision. The Society of Friends does not have an official position on donation.

UNITARIAN UNVERSALIST

Organ and tissue donation is widely supported by Unitarian Universalists. They view it as an act of love and selfless giving.

UNITED CHURCH OF CHRIST

The Director of Washington Office of the United Church of Christ, Reverend Jay Lintner, states: "United Church of Christ people, churches and agencies are extremely and overwhelmingly supportive of organ sharing. The General Synod has never spoken to this issue because, in general, the Synod speaks on more controversial issues, and there is no controversy about organ sharing, just as there is no controversy about blood donation in the denomination. While the General Synod has never spoken about blood donation, blood donation rooms have been set up at several General Synods. Similarly, any organized effort to get the General Synod delegates or individual churches to sign organ donation cards would meet with general positive responses."

UNITED METHODIST

The United Methodist Church issued a policy statement regarding organ and tissue donation. In it, they state that, "The United Methodist

Church recognizes the life-giving benefits of organ and tissue donation, and thereby encourages all Christians to become organ and tissue donors by signing and carrying cards or driver's licenses, attesting to their commitment of such organs upon their death, to those in need, as a part of their ministry to others in the name of Christ, who gave his life what we might have life in its fullness."

Chapter Ten

Bereavement & Care for the Bereaved
Addressing Issues of Loss, Grief, and Bereavement by Health Care Professionals

*For everything there is a season,
and a time for every matter under heaven:
a time to be born, and a time to die;
a time to plant, and a time to pluck up what is planted...(Eccl 3:4-5).*

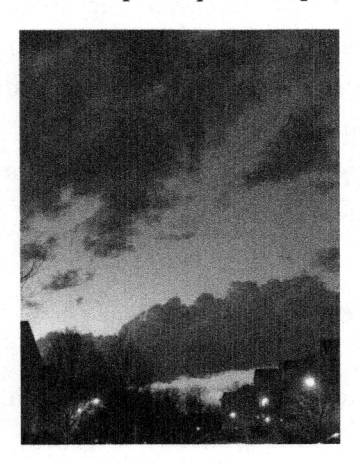

In this chapter, we shall be discussing the following key points:

- ❖ Understand the basic concept of "Bereavement"
- ❖ Discuss the five stages of loss & grief
- ❖ Discuss the common reactions of grief
- ❖ Examine some clinical recommendations for bereavement care
- ❖ Examine some professional guidelines for clinical practice in caring for the bereaved.

What is Bereavement?

What is bereavement? An English dictionary defines "Bereavement" as an incident that leaves someone desolate or alone, especially by death. In an ancient or old-fashioned definition, the word also means "to take something valuable or necessary typically by force." That is, it is considered as a condition of having been deprived of something greatly valued.[166] However, for the purpose of this Book, our working definition of the word "Bereavement" is: a condition of having been deprived or the loss of a family member, a relative, a friend, or a colleague, through death. A bereaved person could suffer brokenness of heart, a sense of shattered heart, and a deep sense of emotional frailties. It is common that bereavement evokes a very deep sense of loss and grief. Loss and Grief are the emotional aftermath of bereavement, which could affect everyone connected with the deceased – families, friends, and the care team – in different ways. Not only that bereavement, loss and grief, occur more often in a healthcare setting; but also, in order to fully understand bereavement fully, it is important to examine Loss & Grief and its stages, and the common reactions to grief, especially in a hospital or a nursing home or any other clinical environment.

What is Loss & Grief?

Grief is defined as the "normal but bewildering cluster of ordinary human emotions arising in response to a significant loss, which can be intensified and complicated by the level of relationship to the person or the object lost."[167] Consequent cluster of emotions that can result from loss and grief are: guilt, shame, loneliness, anxiety, anger, terror, bewilderment, emptiness, profound sadness, despair, and helplessness. All are part of grief and loss, and are common to being humans regardless of external factors that differentiate human race. It is pertinent to note that someone may experience grief and loss, not only after the death of a loved one (bereavement), but it can begin and continue throughout the hospitalization or illness (for patients in nursing facilities, hospice – home or facility).[168]

The Five Stages of Loss & Grief[169]

- ◆ Denial and Isolation
- ◆ Anger
- ◆ Bargaining
- ◆ Depression
- ◆ Acceptance

Stage 1: Denial & Isolation

Isolation is a necessary consequence of loss. It is a collapse of one's world and the erosion of internal self-certainty that require some time of retreat from demanding social interactions. The grieving person feels vulnerable, shrinks from public scrutiny of thoughts and feelings, and thus needs a safe place to be. Isolation creates such a safe place.[170]

This first stage of loss & grief, "Denial and Isolation," the bereaved out-rightly denies the reality of the situation. This stage demonstrates the "normal" human tendency and reaction to rationalize an overwhelming emotional incident, float a defense mechanism that buffers the immediate shock, and thus, enable the bereaved to sustain the wave of emotional pain through the temporary response of denial and isolation.[171] Even when bereavement was anticipated, physicians and the care team should not be surprised that bereaved family display this sense of denial and emotional isolation.

Stage 2: Anger

It is not unusual to display an emotion of anger whenever we are deprived of something or someone of immense value to us. Families, friends or other relations may display some "anger" when their loved one passed, regardless of its suddenness or anticipated. However, a sudden death can aggravate the intensity of the anger, and its expression can be spontaneous. For the bereaved dealing with shock and sudden death of a loved one, both stage 1 and 2 can occur simultaneously, with such expressions as: "No, no, no...it can't be true!" or "We are not ready for this..." It is important for the care team that anger may be "misdirected" at the physician or the nurse or any other employee of the care unit. It can even be redirected at the deceased or family members.

Stage 3: Bargaining

The normal reaction to feelings of helplessness and vulnerability is often a need to regain control, which could be expressed in such words as: "If only we had sought medical attention sooner...," "if only we got a second opinion from another doctor...," "if only we had tried to be there for him or for her..." "If only I had visited sooner..." "If only the doctor had done..." It is not unusual for a bereaved family to express this "bargaining" tendency, especially as the family seeks to "postpone the inevitable."[172]

Stage 4: Depression

Two types of depression are associated with mourning. The first one is a reaction to practical implications relating to the loss. Sadness and regret dominate this type of depression. Often, the bereaved worry, in their grief, that they have spent less time with others who depend who them, perhaps the deceased. For the care team who provide grief support, this phase may be eased by simple clarification, words of reassurance, and a few kind words.

The second type of depression is more subtle and, in a sense, seems more private. It is a quiet preparation to separate and to bid the deceased loved one farewell. Sometimes, what the bereaved needs is a hug.

Stage 5: Acceptance

This phase is marked by withdrawal and calm. The bereaved is able to see the reality of the loss for what it truly is.

Common Grief Reactions

In most clinical environments, or care-providing centers, we are often exposed to reactions from bereaved family members and friends, arising from loss and grief. Hence, it is important to examine some of the possible common reactions of grief. Grief reactions are classified into five different categories: thought patterns (cognitive), physical sensations, emotions, behaviors, and spiritual.[173] We shall briefly examine each of these reactions.

Grief Reactions: Thought Patterns (Cognitive)

Although these are not arranged in any particular order; however, for the purpose of this presentation, the first language of grief is Cognitive reaction. That is, the thought patterns of the bereaved or the grieving persons. This includes confusion or poor concentration, self-blame, disbelief, forgetfulness or problems with short term memory, pre-occupation with thoughts of the deceased, acceptance, lost of sense of purpose, and, shift in perspectives.

- ◈ **Cognitive (Thought Patterns)**
    - ◇ **Disbelief.** This is often our first thought upon hearing of a death, especially if the death was sudden.
    - ◇ **Confusion.** This manifests as having trouble concentrating, being forgetful, and experiencing confused thinking.
    - ◇ **Preoccupation.** We may spend lots of time thinking about the deceased or obsessing about their suffering and dying.
    - ◇ **Sense of the Deceased's Presence.** This is most likely to happen shortly after the death.
    - ◇ **Hallucinations.** It is a fairly common and normal symptom of bereavement to see or hear a loved one, usually within a few weeks after the death.[174]

Grief Reactions: Physical Sensations

For a grieving person experiencing physical sensations, reactions will include symptoms of shock, tightness in chest or forehead or throat, dry mouth, breathlessness or shortness of breath, nausea or hollow feeling in the stomach, weakness or restlessness or lack of energy, disruption to sleeping and eating patterns, hypersensitivity to noise, emptiness, and sense of depersonalization.

- **Physical Sensations**
  - Tightness in the forehead, throat, or chest
  - Dry mouth
  - Breathlessness or shortness of breath
  - Nausea and/or a hollow feeling in the stomach
  - Hypersensitivity to noise
  - Lack of energy, weakness, restlessness
  - Sense of depersonalization[175]

Grief Reactions: Emotions

The emotional grief reaction include numbness, anger, sadness or crying or wailing, helplessness or hopelessness or fear, guilt or relief, despair or feeling lost, calm, overwhelmed, abandoned, free, anxious, frustration or powerlessness, and conflicting emotions.

- **Emotions**
  - Shock. This occurs most often in the case of a sudden death, but may also occur after an expected death.
  - Numbness. This is commonly experienced early in the grieving process and serves to protect us from being overwhelmed by a flood of feelings.

- Sadness. This is the most familiar reaction to grief, and it helps us by evoking sympathy and protective responses in those around us.

- Irritability & Anger: This anger comes from two sources:

- We feel frustrated that we couldn't prevent the death.

- It is a normal regressive experience to feel anger at the person that "abandoned" us.

- These feelings need to be acknowledged. It is very common to displace anger onto another target, such as health care personnel.

- Guilt: Guilt is a very common symptom of bereavement, particularly in the case of a suicide.

- Anxiety: The way of looking at the world may have been shattered by the loss. This can be due to:

- Sense of insecurity (fear of independence),

- Panic attack,

- A heightened sense of one's own mortality.

- Loneliness: This is particularly a problem for surviving spouses. It may be very intense if we had an extremely close relationship.

- Fatigue: Grief is emotionally exhausting. This fatigue can be surprising and distressing to an active person.

- Helplessness, hopelessness, fear: The stress of bereavement is heightened by the fact that there is nothing we can do to reverse the death.

- Yearning, abandoned: Missing the deceased is a normal response to loss. Families and friends express this in different ways.

- Emancipation: This is a positive feeling that may come after a death, particularly in a difficult or highly conflicted relationship.

◈ Relief: Many people feel relief after the death of a loved one, particularly if the loved one suffered during a lengthy illness. Relief is often accompanied by a sense of guilt.[176]

Grief Reactions: Behavioral

Behavioral reactions vary from person to person, culture to culture, and from one social disposition to another. However, most of the behavioral reactions listed in this presentation transcend cultural, racial, or gender boundaries. These include: crying, with or without visible tears; calling out for the deceased by name; pacing or restlessness or display of over activity; social withdrawal or isolation; searching for information or the need for conceptual understanding from different sources; verbal expression of anger, silence, dissociation, or even intermittent display of absent-mindedness. The clinical team, especially the physician, should bear in mind that some of these, especially absent mindedness, could occur in the course of post-demise brief with the bereaved family. Hence, it will be advisable for the physician, leading the family meeting, to speak slowly, repeat key points, pause and allow the family to "absorb" the essentials of the information, as this will help their grief process, and the overall positive outcome of the meeting. Sleep disturbances, as well as obstruction in eating pattern, can be noticeable with family members as they go through grief behavioral reaction, especially when their loved one is actively dying. This grief reaction is often expressed by family members sitting by the bedside of a loved one for several hours, day and night, often time without food or sleep. The clinical team can help grieving family to reduce these disturbances by letting them know the potential risks attached to skipping meals, or not getting some needed hours of rest.

These other grief behavioral reactions – social withdrawal, dreams of the deceased, avoiding reminders of the deceased, and visiting places or carrying objects that remind them of the deceased – often occur outside the clinical setting. However, this can also be expressed when a family member feels not strong enough to see/view a loved one who has just died. Some are not able to behold the presence of a deceased, and some would want to retain a different image other than the dead body image. Suffices to know that these grief behavioral reactions are not strange, and they should not be adjudged as such. Grief is peculiar to an individual's emotional strength, disposition, and the coping level.

- ❖ Behavioral
    - ◇ Crying: There is potential healing value in crying, because our tears release mood altering chemicals.
    - ◇ Searching or Calling Out for the Deceased.
    - ◇ Restless Over-activity.
    - ◇ Sleep Disturbances: These are very common. They may sometimes require medical intervention, but in normal grief they usually correct themselves. They can sometimes symbolize various fears, such as the fear of dreaming, the fear of being in bed alone, and the fear of not wakening up.
    - ◇ Appetite Disturbances: Loss of appetite is more common than increased appetite, but both are very common.
    - ◇ Absent-Minded Behavior: This can happen while receiving the sad news of death.
        - • This can be dangerous if, for example, we are not paying attention while crossing the street or driving.
    - ◇ Social Withdrawal: This is usually short-lived and corrects itself. It can also include a loss of interest in the outside world, i.e., TV, newspapers, etc.
    - ◇ Dreams of the Deceased: Both dreams and nightmares are very common.
    - ◇ Avoiding Reminders of the Deceased: Someone may avoid places or things that trigger painful feelings of grief.
    - ◇ Visiting Places/Carrying Objects that Remind of the Deceased: This is for the fear of losing memories of the deceased.[177]

Grief Reactions: Spiritual

When death occurs, it is not unusual for the bereaved to engage in series of spiritual tendencies. These include blame, whereby the individual attempts to seek justifications or find rational meaningful answers to the loss. Faith and beliefs play huge factor in a grief process or in dealing with sad news of a loss. Faith and belief can become strong pillars of support for the bereaved, thereby yielding positive outcome and strength. Or, it can suffer serious spiritual fracture such as doubts, questions, scars, and so on.

- Spiritual
  - Blame: This is a human tendency to seek a "justification" for the loss, or something to hold-on to.
  - Exploring hope and purpose: Several "*whys?*" are repeatedly asked from the clinical team, seeking possible answers to the loss.
  - Wanting to die or join the deceased: Letting-go can be a huge factor in a grief process.
  - Placement of faith and beliefs
    - Supported and strengthened by faith and beliefs – positive spiritual/emotional reaction/outcome
    - Spiritual/emotional scars – negative spiritual reaction/outcome.[178]

Grief Reactions: Summary[179]

- Despair
- Disbelief
- Denial
- Anger
- Shock
- Inconsolable wailing, tearing of clothing
- Sorrow
- Deep sadness
- Fainting
- Vomiting
- Shortness of breath
- Hyperventilation

- Helplessness
- Guilt
- Cardiac chest pains are also possible physical responses.

Recommendations for Bereavement Care

The following recommendations for bereavement care are provided, based on the recommendations from the Institute of Medicine, the National Comprehensive Cancer Network, and the American College of Chest Physicians' professional, emphasizing the importance of information, education, and sensitivity to cultural differences while providing emotional support to the bereaved.

- Professional tasks following bereavement:
  - Information and education, with sensitivity to what people seem to want to know
  - Emotional support
  - Clinical recognition of abnormal bereavement reactions
  - Legitimization of the occurrence of death, so that the bereaved are assured that all therapeutically/clinically appropriate measures were attempted.

- Professional Obligations following bereavement:
  - The well-being of family is part of the health professional's responsibility when death occurs.
  - Health providers and healthcare institutions have a continuing responsibility to assist the bereaved.
  - Health providers should be aware of variations in grief responses that may occur among family members, based on ethnicity, culture, customs, traditions, etc.
  - Routine history taking in primary care settings should include questions about recent losses, and then, alert Spiritual Care for support.[180]

When Death Occurs: Clinical Practice Guidelines

The death of a loved one can heightened the need for cultural and spiritual sensitivity from the care providers. When death occurs, be sure to follow medical protocols but within the context of cultural and religious practices of the patient and his/her family. When not certain, be sure to inquire from the family if there are any specific cultural and religious practices that the team can provide, in order to assist in their grief process.

When death occurs, as a general rule, kindly offer condolences to the bereaved. If you need to break death news, kindly find a very conducive environment – such as, a place to sit – before you break the news to the family. Also, be prepared to answer questions from the bereaved family (in case they have one). If this is not related to medical cause of death, outside your professional care, do involve the appropriate service team to attend the concerns of the family.

- **Immediate after death care (for family, loved ones & caregivers):**
  - Remove implanted devices, except for death cases to be reviewed by medical examiners.
  - Ensure religious and cultural sensitiveness, and respectful treatment of the body
  - Provide family time and space with the deceased
  - Inform/involve other healthcare professionals to address survivor's concerns (chaplain, social worker, decedent affairs, etc)
  - Offer guidance or normal bereavement process
  - Comfort tray may be helpful, but you may first ask the family as not to be culturally offended.
  - Prepare death certificate, complete forms, and provide necessary information for funeral arrangements - contact decedent affairs personnel.
  - Formally express condolences on patient's death

- Acknowledge the loss

- Attend intentional debriefing meeting with family, especially if the family desires one

- Be empathetic, accept human limitations, and do not be dismissive of concerns or avoidable interjections.

- Refer to appropriate bereavement services within the institution or in the community.[181]

Bereavement Care & Cultural Context

First, everyone experiences grief and loss, but expression of feelings and experiences of loss vary from culture to culture. Secondly, there is neither a universal way nor a correct way to grieve or mourn. In order to be culturally sensitive to the bereaved, you may ask:

- What emotions and behaviors are considered normal grief within the grieving person's culture?

- What are the bereaved family's beliefs around death?

- Is there anything I can do to help?

Remember that not all cultures value comfort trays, gifts, flowers, or similar kind gestures when mourning. Also remember, that a family member is not physically sobbing does not mean he or she is not grieving, and there is no "appropriate" way to grief. In brief, remember these:

- Culture, gender and other factors may affect how grief is felt and expressed – no uniformity.

- Relatives may become silent & withdrawn, deny or become aggressive – reactions varied.

- Research suggests that these extremes can be better managed by clinicians or the care team through these:

    - A comfortable non-denominational venue to ensure privacy;

> Tailored emotional support and honest information (oral and written) relevant to families' needs;

> Providing opportunities for families to verbalize emotions and have questions answered sensitively, simply, clearly, and informatively;

> Providing access to spiritual care;

> Offering relatives opportunities to view the deceased.

> The ***appearance of the deceased*** and how families are treated during such occasions may affect how they cope with their bereavement in the long term.

Dying With Dignity – A Basic Human Right

It is hard to believe that there's someone who doesn't want to die with every sense of human dignity. Sense of dignity would include dying where you'd wanted or at least preferred; to be surrounded by family, friends and loved ones, to breathe the last peacefully and possibly painlessly, and so on. In brief, majority of people suffering from a terminal illness seem to prefer to die at home, rather than in hospital or a hospice, research has shown. For instance, Muslims, like many other ardent believers, would wish to die at home. Making death clinical and remote in a hospital setting is not in keeping with many religious traditions.

A prospective study of the place of death of 160 patients referred to a hospital support team was carried out. Of these patients 62% died in hospital, 26% at home and 12% in a hospice. Overall, 56% of patients (90) were able to express a preference for place of death; 48 patients wished to die at home and 26 wanted to be cared for in a hospice. 71% of these patients achieved their choice but the remainder became too unwell to transfer and died in hospital. From studies, therefore, most patients would prefer to die at home, in the company of families, friends and loved ones.[182]

In order to increase the chances of hospitalized patients to realize their preferred place of final breath of life – to die at home – it is crucial that End-of-Life (EOL) conversations are facilitated in a timely manner. This can help the patient and family embrace the inevitable where they would most prefer. Rather than offering "glimpse of *hope*" or "let's-try-this" syndrome amidst unrealistic goal and the inevitable, clinicians' openness and straightforwardness with patients and caregivers may less complicate the road to a peaceful-die-at-home. The act of "let's-try-this" has sometimes made patients turn out for the worse while the "glimpse of *hope*" initially given to the patient and family disappears in no time. Sometimes, caregivers become angrier when such *hope* is dashed. Perhaps, as some would say, "you'd better let us deal with our situation then than now!" It is important to say, however, that as dicey as patient's situation can be sometimes, one cannot but laud the brilliant efforts of some physicians as they deal with high level of human unpredictability. Suffice it to say that some physicians might offer such *hope* with high sense of sincerity, genuine intention, concern, and unflinching hope that things will work as they expect, within the tenets of medicine and technology.

Since it is more *yea* than *nay* that most people prefer to die in the comfort of their home and among their family and friends, physicians can help dying patients realize this utmost desire by knowing when to stop aggressive care and shift to comfort goal of care – palliative care or hospice care. With this, patients do not become overly sick and unresponsive due to medical procedures or aggressive medical plan that weakens the frailty of the body than the actual cause of illness.

Prayer: 'As I Care'

As I Care for my patients today,
Be there with me, O Lord, I pray
Make my words kind – it means so much –
And in my hands place Your healing touch
Let your love shine through all that I do,
So those in need may hear and feel You.

–Author Unknown.

Anthony Ade Akinlolu

God *of Many Names*

Names, Titles & Phrases for the DEAREST FRIEND
Of those living in the Desert of Illness

All Powerful God
Almighty giver of good
Answer to all mysteries
Awesome God
Awesome One
Binder of Wounds
Brightness of Faithful Soul
Comfort of Sufferers
Companion of the lonely
Creative Source of all Being
Creator and Preserver of all humankind
Creator of all
Creator of goodness and beauty
Creator of the light
Desire of all nations
Eternal Father-Mother-God
Eternal God our answer
Eternal Keeper
Eternal One
Eternal Ruler
God arrayed in justice
God of ages past and future
God of all being
God of all comfort
God of compassion
God of all creatures
God of all fresh
God of all generations
God of all goodness
God of all power
Eternal Source of knowledge
Eternal Source of Peace
Eternal Spirit of the Universe
Ever living God
Ever loving God
Faithful God
The first and the last
Fountain of all Holiness
Fountain of everlasting light
Fountain of life
Fountain of light and truth
Fountain of Wisdom
Friend of the Poor
Generous Provider of good gift
Giver of all good things
Giver of every good and perfect gift
Giver of health and salvation
Giver of life and health
Giver of love
Giver of Peace
God of many deliverances
God of Peace
God of power and splendor
God prophets (and apostles)
God of all righteousness
God of steadfastness and encouragement
God of the beginning, God of the end
God of the loving heart
God of the morning, noon,
    and evening and life

God of all the world
God of all times and places
God of earth and air, height and depth
God of earthquake, wind and fire
God of eternal might
God of forgiveness and understanding
God of freedom and right
God of grace and glory
God of heavenly powers
God of Holiness
God of holy love
God of hope and joy
God of Israel's past
God of life and depth
God of light and Sun
Guardian of our lives
Guide of humanity
Healer of the sick
Heart's Delight
Helper of all persons
Hidden God
(The) Hope of all the ends of the earth
Incognito God
Judge of all humankind
Keeper of our souls
Life of mortal
Life of the world
Light of the faithful
Lover of concord
Lover of souls
Maker of heaven and earth
Maker of man and woman in your own likeness
Mighty Redeemer

God of the spirits of all flesh
God of this day
God of truth
God of unchanging power
God of wonders
God our Companion
God our helper
God surrounded by glory
God who art perfect love
Gracious giver of knowledge
Gracious God
Great God (of power)
Great God our Hope
Great Ruler of the world
Great Healer of body and soul
Guide of the Meek
Guide and inspiration of humanity
Heart that inspires in us a vision justice and love
Helper of the weak
High and Holy One
Judge Eternal
Inexhaustible God
Inspiration of goodness
Keeper of (the) covenant(s)
Life of all who live
Life of the universe
Life of all seeing
Light of the minds that know thee
Lover of peace
Maker of all things
Maker of light
Mighty forever God
Mighty God
Mind of the universe

(The) Mind that unifies all creation
One and Eternal of time and space
Our Creator and Out Teacher
Our Source and Our End
Power that saves
Power that shields
Protector of all who trust
Radiance of faithful souls
Redeemer and Deliverer
Redeemer of the oppresses
Refuge of those who put their trust in you
Righteous One of all generations
Rock of Jacob
Ruler of all people on earth
Ruler of the universe
Shelter from the storm
Shield of our fathers and mothers
Source of all existence
Source of all power
Source of all true joy
Source of creation
Source of eternal light
Source Good
Source of life
Source of peace
Source of salvation
Source of truth and law
Sovereign of peace
Steadfast and loving one
Strength of the weak
Strong God of truth
Sustainer of all the worlds that are
True and only light
Watchful and caring God

Most merciful God
Only one
Our Refuge and Our Strength
(The) Power that brings healing to the sick
Proclaimer of Justice
Pure and upright one
Radiant and glorious God
Redeemer of Israel
Redeeming God
Repose of dead
Righteous God
Rock of all creation
Rock of our life
Ruler of all creation
Searcher of hearts
Shield of Abraham
Shining Glory
Source of all health
Source of all that we have and are
Source of blessing
Sources of deliverance and help
Source of freedom
Source of good and strength
Source of life
Source of mercy
Source of strength
Sovereign God
Staff and support of the righteous
Strength of our life
Strength of those who labor
Support of the innocent
Teacher of peace
True sun of the world
(The) Will that gives us power

Upholder of the falling	World's Light
Wondrous Fashioner and
   Sustainer of life

Source: NCCC. (1984). Language and the Church: Designs for Workshops.

Endnotes

1. Amenta, M.O. (1986). Spiritual Concerns (Chapter 9, pp. 115 – 161). In M.O. Amenta & N. Bohnet (Eds.). *Nursing care of the terminally ill*. Boston: Little, Brown.
2. Susan Wintz, Earl Cooper. (2009). *Cultural & Spiritual Sensitivity: A learning module for health care professionals.*
3. Stoll, R.I. (1989). The essence of spirituality. In V.B. Carson (Ed.). *Spiritual Dimensions of Nursing Practice* (pp. 4-23). Philadelphia: Saunders.
4. Tanyi, R.A. (2002). Towards clarification of the meaning of spirituality. *Journal of Advanced Nursing*, 39(5), 500-9.
5. Karin Kolsky, 'Spiritual Issues' in End-of-Life. Maryland: National Institute on Aging.
6. Reed, P. (1992). An emerging paradigm for the investigation of spirituality in nursing. *Research in Nursing & Health, 15,* 349-357.
7. David F. Kelly (2004). *Contemporary Catholic Health Care Ethics*. Washington, D.C.: Georgetown University Press.
8. Wintz and Cooper, 2009.
9. Mauk, Kristen L., Schmidt, Nola K. (2004). *Spiritual Care in Nursing Practice*. Philadelphia: Lippincott Williams & Wilkins; Burkhardt, M.A., & Jacobson, M. G. N. (2000). Spirituality and health. In B. M. Dossey, L. Keegan, & C. E. Guzzetta (Eds.), *Holistic nursing: A handbook for practice* (3rd ed., pp. 91-121); Stoll, R. I. (1989). The essence of spirituality. In V. B. Carson (Ed.), *Spiritual dimensions of nursing practice* (pp. 4-23) Philadelphia: W. B. Saunders.
10. John Patton. (2005). *Pastoral Care: An Essential Guide.* Nashville: Abingdon Press
11. K.C. Brownstone, "Pastoral Care of Dying" http://ezinearticles.com Retrieved March 15, 2011
12. David F. Kelly (2004) Contemporary Catholic Health Care Ethics.
13. Remen R. Naomi. (2006). *Kitchen Table Wisdom: Stories that Heal*. New York:

The Penguin Group. Pp.219-220
14. Remen, R. N. (2006). *Kitchen Table Wisdom: Stories that Heal*. New York: The Penguin Group. P.220
15. Fowler, M., & Peterson, B.S. (1997). Spiritual themes in clinical pastoral education. *Journal of Training and Supervision in Ministry*, 18, 46-54
16. Dossey, B.M., & Guzzetta, C.E. (2000). Holistic nursing practice. In B.M. Dossey, L. Keegan, & C.E. Guzzetta (Eds.), *Holistic nursing: A handbook for practice* (3rd ed., pp. 5-26), Rockville, MD: Aspen.
17. Doehring, Carrie. (2006). *The Practice of Pastoral Care: A Postmodern Approach*. Kentucky: Westminster John Knox Press.
18. Doehring, Carrie. (2006). *The Practice of Pastoral Care: A Postmodern Approach*.
19. John E. Babler, "A Comparison of Spiritual Care Provided by Social Workers, Nurses, and Spiritual Care Professionals," *The Hospice Journal*, 1997, Vol. 12, No. 4, pp. 15-28 as quoted by Kathleen Galek, Ph.D. *et al*, "Spiritual Needs: Gender Differences among Professional Spiritual Care Providers," *The Journal of Pastoral Care & Counseling*, Vol. 62, Nos. 1-2, Spring-Summer 2008, pg 29
20. Remen, R. N. (2006). *Kitchen Table Wisdom: Stories that Heal*. New York: The Penguin Group. P. 144
21. Remen, R. N. (2006). *Kitchen Table Wisdom: Stories that Heal*. P. 144
22. This Chapter was first presented at a Community Clergy Intensive Workshop hosted by MedStar Washington Hospital Center Community Clergy Institute, September 21-23, 2011.
23. Louis Nieuwenhuizen, "Spiritual Care Illustrated: Creating a Shared Language" *The Journal of Pastoral Care & Counseling*, 2007, Vol. 61
24. Louis Nieuwenhuizen, "Spiritual Care Illustrated: Creating a Shared Language" *The Journal of Pastoral Care & Counseling*, 2007, Vol. 61
25. M.R. Telfer and J.P. Sheperd, "Psychological Stress in Patients...," International *Journal of Oral Maxillofacial Surgery*, 1993, Vol. 22, pp. 347-349; M.G. Tilter, M.Z. Cohen, & M.J. Craft,
26. Louis Nieuwenhuizen, "Spiritual Care Illustrated: Creating a Shared Language", *The Journal of Pastoral Care & Counseling*, 2007, Vol. 61, No.4, pp.329-341
27. Stoll, R.I. (1983). Emotional and spiritual support. In T.C. Kravis & C.G. Warner (Eds.). *Emergency medicine: A comprehensive review*. Rockville, MD: Aspen; Dombeck, M.B. (1996). Chaos and self-organization as a consequence

of spiritual disequilibrium. *Clinical Nurse Specialist*. 10(2), 69-75.
28. North American Nursing Diagnosis Association (NANDA), 1999-2000
29. Taylor, Elizabeth J. (2002). *Spiritual Care: Nursing Theory, Research, and Practice*. New Jersey: Pearson Education, Inc.
30. Mako C, Galek K, Poppito SR: Spiritual pain among patients with advanced cancer in palliative care. Journal of Palliative Medicine 2006 Oct; 9(5):1106-13.
31. North American Nursing Diagnosis Association (NANDA), 1999-2000
32. NANDA, 2000
33. Gover, I. (2000). Spiritual care in nursing: A systematic approach. *Nursing Standard*, 14, 32-40; Taylor, Elizabeth J. (2002). *Spiritual Care: Nursing Theory, Research, and Practice*; Ferrell B. R. (1996). *Suffering*. Boston: Jones & Bartlett.
34. Balboni TA, Vanderwerker LC, Block SD, et al.: Religiousness and spiritual support among advanced cancer patients and associations with end-of-life treatment preferences and quality of life. Journal Clinical Oncology 2007 Feb 10; 25(5):555-60.
35. "Average U.S. ER wait time 4-plus hours" Health News, United Press International, UPI.com, published: July 26, 2010. Retrieved July 23, 2012 http://www.upi.com/Health_News/2010/07/26/Average-US-ER-wait-time-4-plus-hours/UPI-76891280122494/
36. Todd Neale, "Fast Treatment Rare in Emergency Departments, Survey Says" July 25, 2010. ABC News http://abcnews.go.com/Health/Wellness/er-wait-times-longer-survey/story?id=11240084
37. Todd Neale, "Fast Treatment Rare in Emergency Departments, Survey Says" July 25, 2010
38. Todd Neale, "Fast Treatment Rare in Emergency Departments, Survey Says" July 25, 2010.
39. James Ball and Denis Campbell, "NHS waiting times increase for diagnostic tests" July 6, 2011 http://www.guardian.co.uk/society/2011/jul/06/nhs-waiting-times-increase-diagnostic-tests Retrieved July 23, 2012
40. James Ball and Denis Campbell, "NHS waiting times increase for diagnostic tests" July 6, 2011
41. Bob Doherty, "Wait Times For Medical Care: How the US Actually Measures Up" Better Health Network, Health Policy. February 2, 2010 http://getbetterhealth.com/wait-times-for-medical-care-how-the-us-actually-

measures-up/2010.02.02 Retrieved July 23, 2012

42. Margarita. "Long Doctor Visit? Average Patient Wait Time Creeps Up To 21.3 Minutes" November 17, 2009 http://spotlight.vitals.com/2009/11/long-doctor-visit-average-patient-wait-time-creeps-up-to-213-mins Retrieved July 23, 2012

43. David C. Johnson, BCC. Presidential Address, June 23, 2012 APC Conference Member Recognition Luncheon APC e-News July, 2012 – Vol. 14 No. 5

44. *This talk was delivered by theologian Hans Küng March 31, 2005, at the opening of the Exhibit on the World's Religions at Santa Clara University. The exhibit was prepared by the Global Ethic Foundation, of which Kung is co-founder and president. Source: http://www.scu.edu/ethics/practicing/focusareas/global_ethics/laughlin-lectures/kung-world-religions.html*

45. Interfaith International (2008). http://www.interfaithonline.org/

46. "'Doctor, will you pray with me?': Chicago Conference Addresses How Physicians Should Respond" Advisory Board Company, June 11, 2012. Retrieved August 1, 2012 http://www.advisoryboardcompany.com/Daily-Briefing/2012/06/11/Doctor-will-you-pray-with-me

47. "'Doctor, will you pray with me?': Chicago Conference Addresses How Physicians Should Respond" Advisory Board Company, June 11, 2012. Retrieved August 1, 2012 http://www.advisoryboardcompany.com/Daily-Briefing/2012/06/11/Doctor-will-you-pray-with-me

48. "'Doctor, will you pray with me?': Chicago Conference Addresses How Physicians Should Respond" Advisory Board Company, June 11, 2012. Retrieved August 1, 2012 http://www.advisoryboardcompany.com/Daily-Briefing/2012/06/11/Doctor-will-you-pray-with-me

49. Johnson, E. E. (2006). This is about difference. *The Journal of Pastoral Care & Counseling*, 311-314.

50. Barrett, D. J. (2011). *Leadership Communication.* New York: McGraw-Hill/Irwin.

51. Spencer-Oatey, H. (2000). *Culturally Speaking: Mananging Rapport through Talk across Cultures.* London: Continuum.

52. Lehman, D., Fenza, P., & Hollinger-Smith, L. (2001, May). *Diversity & Cultural Competency in Health Care Settings.* Retrieved from Mather LifeWays: www.matherlifeways.com

53. Wells, M. (2000). Beyond cultural competence: A model for individual and institutional cultural development. *Journal for Community Health Nurses*, 189-99.
54. Fleming, M., & Towey, K. (2001). Delivering culturally effective health care to adolescents. *American Medial Association*.
55. Lehman, D., Fenza, P., & Hollinger-Smith, L. (2001, May). *Diversity & Cultural Competency in Health Care Settings*.
56. Committee on Health Care for Underserved Women. (2011, May). *Cultural Sensitivity and Awareness in the Delivery of Health Care*. Retrieved from The American Congress of Obstetricians and Gynecologists: http://www.acog.org/Resources-And-PublicationsCommittee-Opinions/Committee-on-He...
57. Bond, B. (2010, October 6). *Dose of cultural sensitivity helpful in health care setting*. Retrieved from statesman: http://www.statesman.com/news/classifieds/jobs/dose-of-cultural-sensitivity-helpful-in-health...
58. Bond, B. (2010, October 6). *Dose of cultural sensitivity helpful in health care setting*. Retrieved from statesman: http://www.statesman.com/news/classifieds/jobs/dose-of-cultural-sensitivity-helpful-in-health...
59. Lehman, D., Fenza, P., & Hollinger-Smith, L. (2001, May). *Diversity & Cultural Competency in Health Care Settings*.
60. Lehman, D., Fenza, P., & Hollinger-Smith, L. (2001, May). *Diversity & Cultural Competency in Health Care Settings*.
61. Lehman, D., Fenza, P., & Hollinger-Smith, L. (2001, May). *Diversity & Cultural Competency in Health Care Settings*.
62. Lehman, D., Fenza, P., & Hollinger-Smith, L. (2001, May). *Diversity & Cultural Competency in Health Care Settings*.
63. Lehman, D., Fenza, P., & Hollinger-Smith, L. (2001, May). *Diversity & Cultural Competency in Health Care Settings*.
64. O'Hara-Devereaux, M., & Johansen, R. (1994). *Globalwork: Bridging Distance, Culture, and Time*. San Francisco: Jossey-Bass.
65. Barrett, Deborah J. (2011). *Leadership Communication*.
66. Barrett, Deborah J. (2011). *Leadership Communication*
67. Barrett, Deborah J. (2011). *Leadership Communication*
68. Barrett, Deborah J. (2011). *Leadership Communication*
69. Condon, J.C. (1975). *An Introduction to Intercultural Communication*. New York: Macmillan.

70. Hall, E. T. (1959). *The Silent Language.* Westport, CT: Greenwood Press.
71. Lehman, D., Fenza, P., & Hollinger-Smith, L. (2001, May). *Diversity & Cultural Competency in Health Care Settings.*
72. Fernandez, V. M., & Fernandez, K. M. (1999). *Transcultural Nursing: Basic Concepts and Case Studies.* Retrieved April 06, 2015, from www.megalink.net
73. Fernandez, V. M., & Fernandez, K. M. (1999). *Transcultural Nursing: Basic Concepts and Case Studies.* Retrieved April 06, 2015, from www.megalink.net
74. Gover, I. (2000). Spiritual care in nursing: A systematic approach. *Nursing Standard*, 14, 32-40;
75. per survey published April 28, 2010
76.
77. RCN Survey, 2010
78. "History of Healthcare Chaplaincy and HCMA" http://www.hcmachaplains.org/home/history.html Retrieved July 19, 2012
79. "History of Healthcare Chaplaincy and HCMA" http://www.hcmachaplains.org/home/history.html Retrieved July 19, 2012
80. "History of Healthcare Chaplaincy and HCMA" http://www.hcmachaplains.org/home/history.html Retrieved July 19, 2012
81. "History of Healthcare Chaplaincy and HCMA" http://www.hcmachaplains.org/home/history.html
82. History of Healthcare Chaplaincy and HCMA" http://www.hcmachaplains.org/home/history.html Retrieved July 19, 2012
83. W. Gibson, *A Social History of the Domestic Chaplain, 1530-1840 (London, UK: Leicester University Press, 1997)*, 1-6.
84. "History of Healthcare Chaplaincy and HCMA" Healthcare Chaplains Ministry Association (HCMA) http://www.hcmachaplains.org/home/history.html Retrieved July 19, 2012
85. This work was first published under the title "Holistic healing: At the root of the interdisciplinary team" by *Vision*, National Association of Catholic Chaplains (NACC), Vol. 22, No. 2 March/April, 2012 http://www.nacc.org/vision/Mar_Apr_2012/team-akinlolu.asp
86. This work was also published by *Vision*, National Association of Catholic Chaplains, as a side-bar article under the title "Pastoral Care 'triggers':

Helping Colleagues know when to call the chaplain." Vol. 22, No. 2 March/ April, 2012 http://www.nacc.org/vision/Mar_Apr_2012/team-akinlolu.asp

[87] "Brain Aneurysm - Topic Overview" http://www.webmd.com/brain/tc/brain-aneurysm-topic-overview?page=2 Retrieved August 10, 2012

[88] Remen, R. N. (2006). *Kitchen Table Wisdom: Stories that Heal*. New York: The Penguin Group. P. 52

[89] Mauk & Schmidt, 2004

[90] Lyndon, 2007; Gaffney, 2007; McClelland, 2007; Zboril-Benson, 2002; Schaffner, 2006; Kenyon et al., 2007; Mayo & Duncan, 2004

[91] Baranowsky, A. B. (2002). The silencing response in clinical practice. In C. R. Figley (Ed.). *Treating compassion fatigue*. New York: Brunner-Routledge.

[92] Remen, R. N. (2006). *Kitchen Table Wisdom: Stories that Heal*. New York: The Penguin Group. P. 52

[93] Remen, R. N. (2006). *Kitchen Table Wisdom: Stories that Heal.* P. 54

[94] Mauk, Kristen L., Schmidt, Nola K. (2004). *Spiritual Care in Nursing Practice*. Philadelphia: Lippincott Williams & Wilkins.

[95] Remen, R. N. (2006). *Kitchen Table Wisdom: Stories that Heal.* P. 54

[96] Mauk & Schmidt, 2004

[97] Pfifferling & Gilley, 2000

[98] "World's Top 10 Killer Diseases" http://www.bukisa.com/articles

[99] Steven Reinberg, "Cancer Killed Almost 8 Million Worldwide in 2007" U.S. News & World Report. Posted 12/17/07, Retrieved 06/26/12 http://health.usnews.com/usnews/health/healthday/071217/cancer-killed-almost-8-million-worldwide-in-2007.htm

[100] Charles Patrick Davis, "Cancer" http://www.medicinenet.com/cancer/article.htm Retrieved on June 26, 2012

[101] Charles Patrick Davis, "Cancer" http://www.medicinenet.com/cancer/article.htm Retrieved on June 26, 2012

[102] Kim Y, Wellisch DK, Spillers RL, et al.: Psychological distress of female cancer caregivers: effects of type of cancer and caregivers' spirituality. Support Care Cancer 15 (12): 1367-74, 2007. See also Whitford HS, Olver IN, Peterson MJ: Spirituality as a core domain in the assessment of quality of life in oncology. Psychooncology 17 (11): 1121-8, 2008.

[103] King DE, Bushwick B: Beliefs and attitudes of hospital inpatients about faith healing and prayer. The Journal of Family Practice. 1994 Oct; 39(4):349-52.

Retrieved from http://www.ncbi.nlm.nih.gov on June 26, 2012

[104] Astrow AB, Wexler A, Texeira K, et al.: Is failure to meet spiritual needs associated with cancer patients' perceptions of quality of care and their satisfaction with care? Journal of Clinical Oncology 2007 Dec 20; 25(36):5753-7.

[105] Bowie J, Sydnor KD, Granot M: Spirituality and care of prostate cancer patients: a pilot study. Journal of the National Medical Association 2003 Oct; 95(10):951-4.

[106] Halstead M.T. & Taylor, E.J. (2005). "Spiritual Issues for Cancer Patients" Spiritual Care SIG ToolKit http://wwwnew.towson.edu/sct/connecting.htm

[107] Christina Puchalski, M.D. and Anna L. Romer, Ed.D; Journal of Palliative Medicine Volume 3, Number 1, 2000 Pgs 129 – 137 See also Spiritual Assessment in Clinical Practice, Christina Puchalski, Psychiatric annals; Mar 2006; 36, 3 Psychology Module pg 150

[108] Hallenbeck, James L. (2003). Palliative Care Perspectives. Oxford Press, Inc.

[109] Karen Skalla, "Spiritual Assessment" (2005) Spiritual Care SIG Toolkit http://wwwnew.towson.edu/sct/assessment.htm

[110] Burkhardt, M. A., & Nagai-Jacobson, M. G. (2002). *Spirituality: Living our connectedness*. Albany, NY: Delmar.

[111]

[112] "A Hope and a Prayer for Cancer Patients" beliefnet.com Retrieved June 28, 2012 http://www.beliefnet.com/Health/2005/12/A-Hope-And-A-Prayer-For-Cancer-Patients.aspx

[113] Remen, R. N. (2006). *Kitchen Table Wisdom: Stories that Heal.* P. 65

[114] Remen, R. N. (2006). *Kitchen Table Wisdom: Stories that Heal.* P. 65

[115] Taylor, E. J. (2003). Nurses Caring for the Spirit: Patients with Cancer and Family Caregiver Expectations, *Oncology Nursing Forum, 30,* 585-590.

[116] Halstead M.T. and Taylor, E.J. (2005). "Spiritual Issues for Cancer Patients" Spiritual Care SIG ToolKit http://wwwnew.towson.edu/sct/connecting.htm

[117] Tarumi, Y., Taube, A., Wantanabe, S. (2003). Clinical pastoral education: A physician's experience and reflection on the meaning of spiritual care in palliative care. *The Journal of Pastoral Care and Counseling, 57,* 27-31.

[118] Caron, P. (2005) "Meaning and Purpose" Spiritual Care Special Interest Group Toolkit Project http://wwwnew.towson.edu/sct/meaning%20and%20purpose.htm Retrieved June 28, 2012

[119] Rumbold, B.D. (2003). Caring for the spirit: lessons from working with the dying. *Medical Journal of Australia, 179*(6 Suppl), S11-S13

[120] Viktor Frankl. (1984). Man's Search for Meaning. New York, NY: Simon & Schuster.

[121] St. Thomas Aquinas, Summa IIa IIae, q. 1, a.1, trans. Paul J. Glenn, A Tour of the Summa of St. Thomas Aquinas. (1993). Bangalore: Theological Publications in India.

[122] St. Thomas Aquinas, Summa IIa IIae, q. 1, aa. 4-5

[123] St. Thomas Aquinas: *Quaestiones disputatae de veritate*, q. 14, a.2 ("On faith") Translated by Alfred J. Freddoso, University of Notre Dame. http://www.nd.edu/~afreddos/translat/aquinas5.htm Retrieved August 13, 2012

[124] St. Thomas Aquinas: *Quaestiones disputatae de veritate*, q. 14, a.2 ("On faith") Translated by Alfred J. Freddoso, University of Notre Dame. http://www.nd.edu/~afreddos/translat/aquinas5.htm Retrieved August 13, 2012

[125] Halstead M.T. & Taylor, E.J. (2005). "Spiritual Issues for Cancer Patients" Spiritual Care SIG ToolKit http://wwwnew.towson.edu/sct/connecting.htm

[126] Halstead M.T. & Taylor, E.J. (2005). "Spiritual Issues for Cancer Patients" Spiritual Care SIG ToolKit http://wwwnew.towson.edu/sct/connecting.htm

[127] Azim Khamisa & Jillian Quinn. "The Journey to Forgiveness" Institute for Spirituality & Wellness. http://www.ctschicago.edu/index.php/mnuacademicprograms/cts-centers/261-journey-to-forgiveness. Retrieved on July 1 2012

[128] As Referenced by Azim Khamisa & Jillian Quinn. "The Journey to Forgiveness" Institute for Spirituality & Wellness

[129] Cassell, E. J. (1991). *The nature of suffering*. New York: Oxford University Press.

[130] Kahn, D. L., & Steeves, R. H. (1986). The experience of suffering: Conceptual clarification and theoretical definition. *Journal of Advanced Nursing*, 11, 623-631.

[131] National Cancer Institute, "Understanding Chemotherapy" http://www.cancer.gov/cancertopics/coping/chemo-side-effects Retrieved July 12, 2012

[132] Taylor, E. J. (1993). Factors associated with meaning in life among people with recurrent cancer. *Oncology Nursing Forum, 20*, 1399-1407.

[133] Susie Steiner, "Top five regrets of the dying" posted Wednesday 1 February 2012 Retrieved July 12, 2012 http://www.guardian.co.uk/lifeandstyle/2012/

feb/01/top-five-regrets-of-the-dying
[134] "Life, Death and Mourning" Jewish Virtual Library, 2012. http://www.jewishvirtuallibrary.org/jsource/Judaism/death.html
[135] "Life, Death and Mourning" Jewish Virtual Library, 2012. http://www.jewishvirtuallibrary.org/jsource/Judaism/death.html
[136] "Life, Death and Mourning" Jewish Virtual Library, 2012. http://www.jewishvirtuallibrary.org/jsource/Judaism/death.html
[137] "Life, Death and Mourning" Jewish Virtual Library, 2012. http://www.jewishvirtuallibrary.org/jsource/Judaism/death.html
[138] Ven. Pende Hawter, "Death and Dying in the Tibetan Buddhist Tradition" http://www.buddhanet.net/deathtib.htm Retrieved July 16, 2012
[139] Ven. Pende Hawter, "Death and Dying in the Tibetan Buddhist Tradition"
[140] Susan Thrane, "Hindu End of Life Death, Dying, Suffering, and Karma" Journal of Hospice and Palliative Nursing November/December 2010, Vol. 12 No. 6 Pages 337 – 342 Citing So, how many Hindus are there in the US? *Hinduism Today*. 2008:61 & Hindu American Foundation. Hindu demographics. Hindu American Foundation 2009; http://www.hafsite.org/resources/hinduism_101?q=resources/hinduism_101/hinduism_. Accessed November 12, 2009.
[141] Subramuniyaswami SS. Hinduism, the greatest religion in the world. *What Is Hinduism?* Kapaa, HI: Himalayan Academy; 2007:4-19
[142] Subramuniyaswami SS. Hinduism, the greatest religion in the world. *What Is Hinduism?* Kapaa, HI: Himalayan Academy; 2007:4-19
[143] Subramuniyaswami SS. Hinduism, the greatest religion in the world. *What Is Hinduism?* Kapaa, HI: Himalayan Academy; 2007:4-19
[144] Jeste DV, Vahia IV. Comparison of the conceptualization of wisdom in ancient Indian literature with modern views: focus on the Bhagavad Gita. *Psychiatry Fall*. 2008; 71(3):197-209.
[145] Susan Thrane, "Hindu End of Life Death, Dying, Suffering, and Karma" Journal of Hospice and Palliative Nursing November/December 2010, Vol. 12 No. 6 Pages 337 - 342
[146] Susan Thrane, "Hindu End of Life Death, Dying, Suffering, and Karma" Journal of Hospice and Palliative Nursing November/December 2010, Vol. 12 No. 6 Pages 337 - 342
[147] Whitman SM. Pain and suffering as viewed by the Hindu religion. *J Pain*.

2007; 8(8):607-613.

[148] Susan Thrane, "Hindu End of Life Death, Dying, Suffering, and Karma" Journal of Hospice and Palliative Nursing November/December 2010, Vol. 12 No. 6 Pages 337 - 342

[149] Subramuniyaswami SS. "Ashima: to do no harm". *Hinduism Today*. 2007; 29(1):29-32.

[150] Hinduism Today. Medical ethics. *What Is Hinduism?* Kapaa, HI: Himalayan Academy; 2007:350-357.

[151] Susan Thrane, "Hindu End of Life Death, Dying, Suffering, and Karma" Journal of Hospice and Palliative Nursing November/December 2010, Vol. 12 No. 6 Pages 337 - 342

[152] Hinduism Today. Medical ethics. *What Is Hinduism?* Kapaa, HI: Himalayan Academy; 2007:350-357

[153] Susan Thrane, "Hindu End of Life Death, Dying, Suffering, and Karma" Journal of Hospice and Palliative Nursing November/December 2010, Vol. 12 No. 6 Pages 337 - 342

[154] Field M, Cassell C. Approaching death: improving care at the end of life. (IOM Report) Washington DC: National Academy Press; 1997.

[155] University of Pennsylvania Health System, "Faith Traditions and Health Care" June 2003

[156] Martha R. Jacobs, A Clergy Guide to End-of-Life Issues. 2010. *The Pilgrim Press*. Pp. 88-90

[157] Fazlur Rahman, *Health and Medicine in the Islamic Tradition*, The Crossroad Publishing Company, 1989, pp. 100-129

[158] Aziz Sheikh, "Death and dying – a Muslim perspective," *Journal of the Royal Society of Medicine*, vol 91, March 1998, pp. 138-140

[159] Fazlur Rahman, *Health and Medicine in the Islamic Tradition*

[160] Huda, About.com.Islam, "Islamic Funeral Rites: Care for the dying, funeral prayers, burial, and mourning

[161] Aziz Sheikh, "Death and dying – a Muslim perspective," *Journal of the Royal Society of Medicine*, vol 91, March 1998, pp. 138-140

[162] Fazlur Rahman, Health and Medicine in the Islamic Tradition, The Crossroad Publishing Company, 1989, pp. 100-129

[163] University of Pennsylvania Health System, "Faith Traditions and Health Care" June 2003

[164] University of Pennsylvania Health System, "Faith Traditions and Health Care" June 2003

[165] This is adapted from "Religious Views on Organ, Tissue and Blood Donation" http://www.donatelifenm.org Retrieved on March 14, 2011

[166] "Bereave" http://www.thefreedictionary.com/bereavement

[167] Mitchell, K.R, Anderson, H. (1983). *All our Losses, All our Griefs: Resource for Pastoral Care.* Louisville: Westminster John Knox Press.

[168] INCTR Palliative Care Handbook. (2013).

[169] Kubler-Ross, E (1969). *On Death and Dying*, as used by Axelrod, J. (2006). *The 5 Stages of Loss and Grief*, Retrieved on September 11, 2013, from http://psychcentral.com/lib/the-5-stages-of-loss-and-grief/000617

[170] *Mitchell, K.R., Anderson, H. (1983). All Our Losses, All Our Griefs; The 5 Stages of Loss and Grief*, Retrieved on September 11, 2013, from http://psychcentral.com/lib/the-5-stages-of-loss-and-grief/000617

[171] *Mitchell, K.R., Anderson, H. (1983). All Our Losses, All Our Griefs; The 5 Stages of Loss and Grief,*

[172] Kubler-Ross, E. (1969). *On Death and Dying*, as used by Axelrod, J. (2006). *The 5 Stages of Loss and Grief*, Retrieved on September 11, 2013, from http://psychcentral.com/lib/the-5-stages-of-loss-and-grief/000617

[173] Crisis Support Services of Alameda County "Common Grief Reactions" (2013). http://www.crisissupport.org/grief/common_reactions

[174] Crisis Support Services of Alameda County "Common Grief Reactions" (2013).

[175] Crisis Support Services of Alameda County "Common Grief Reactions" (2013).

[176] Crisis Support Services of Alameda County "Common Grief Reactions" (2013).

[177] Crisis Support Services of Alameda County "Common Grief Reactions" (2013).

[178] Crisis Support Services of Alameda County "Common Grief Reactions" (2013).

[179] Pattison (2008) as used by Marika Hills, et al (2010) "After death 1: caring for bereaved relatives and being aware of cultural differences" in Nursing Times.net

[180] Emanuel et al (2011). "The Role of the Health Professional in Addressing

Issues of Loss, Grief, and Bereavement Experienced by Cancer Patients and Their Families: Managing Reactions to Loss, Grief, and Bereavement"

[181] Emanuel et al (2011). "The Role of the Health Professional in Addressing Issues of Loss, Grief, and Bereavement Experienced by Cancer Patients and Their Families

[182] University of Pennsylvania Health System, "Faith Traditions and Health Care" June 2003

References & Consulted Works

Barrett, D. J. (2011). *Leadership Communication*. New York: McGraw-Hill/Irwin.

Bond, B. (2010, October 6). *Dose of cultural sensitivity helpful in health care setting*. Retrieved from statesman: http://www.statesman.com/news/classifieds/jobs/dose-of-cultural-sensitivity-helpful-in-health...

Burkhardt, M.A., & Jacobson, M. G. N. (2000). Spirituality and health. In B. M. Dossey, L. Keegan, & C. E. Guzzetta (Eds.), *Holistic nursing: A handbook for practice* (3rd ed., pp. 91-121).

Committee on Health Care for Underserved Women. (2011, May). *Cultural Sensitivity and Awareness in the Delivery of Health Care*. Retrieved from The American Congress of Obstetricians and Gynecologists: http://www.acog.org/Resources-And-PublicationsCommittee-Opinions/Committee-on-He...

Donald R. Hands and Wayne L. Fehr, *Spiritual Wholeness for Clergy: A New Psychology of Intimacy with God, Self and Others*, The Alban Institute, 1993, pp. 50-65

Fernandez, V., & Fernandez, K. (1999). *Transcultural Nursing: Basic Concepts and Case Studies*. Retrieved April 06, 2015, from www.megalink.net

Fleming, M., & Towey, K. (2001). Delivering culturally effective health care to adolescents. *American Medial Association*.

John E. Babler, "A Comparison of Spiritual Care Provided by Social Workers, Nurses, and Spiritual Care Professionals," *The Hospice Journal*, 1997

Louis Nieuwenhuizen, "Spiritual Care Illustrated: Creating a Shared Language",

M.R. Telfer and J.P. Sheperd, "Psychological Stress in Patients…," International *Journal of Oral Maxillofacial Surgery*, 1993, Vol. 22, pp. 347-349; M.G. Tilter, M.Z. Cohen, & M.J. Craft, "Impact of Adult Critical Care Hospitalization: Perceptions of Patients, Spouses, Children, and Nurses," Heart Lung, 1991, Vol. 20, No. 2, pp. 174-182; N. Pattison, "Psychological Implications of Admission to Critical Care," British Journal of Nursing, 2005, Vol. 14, No. 13, pp. 708-714; J.E. Rattray, M. Johnson, & J.A. Wildsmith, "Predictors of Emotional Outcomes of Intensive Care," Anaesthesia, 2005, Vol. 60, No. 11, pp. 1085-1092; Louis Nieuwenhuizen, "Spiritual Care Illustrated: Creating a Shared Language", *The Journal of Pastoral Care & Counseling*, 2007, Vol. 61, No.4, pp.329-341

R. Van Pelt, Intensive Care: Helping Teenagers in Crisis (Grand Rapids, MI: Zondervan Publishing House, 1997)

Kent, Carol. (2007). A New Kind of Normal. Tennessee: Thomas Nelson.

Doehring, Carrie. (2006). The Practice of Pastoral Care: A Postmodern Approach. Kentucky: Westminster John Knox Press.

Ronald H. Sunderland. "The Dignity of Servanthood in Pastoral Care" The Journal of Pastoral Care & Counseling, Fall 2003, Vol. 57, No. 3

Subramanina T. "Impact of hospitalization on patients and their families." T. B. Research Center, I.C.M.R., Madras. Indian J Public Health. 1998 Jan-Mar; 42(1):15-6 http://www.ncbi.nlm.nih.gov/pubmed/10389500 Retrieved June 17, 2012

Glaus, 1998; North American Nursing Diagnosis Association, 1996.

Mitchell, K.R, Anderson, H. (1983). *All our Losses, All our Griefs: Resource for Pastoral Care*. Louisville: Westminster John Knox Press.

Stewart, Hays & Ware, 1992.

'What do I say?': Elizabeth Johnston Taylor, Templeton Foundation Press 2007 EOL care for the hospitalized patient. Steven Z. Pantilat MD, Margartet

Isaac MD; Med Clin N Am (2008) 349 – 370

Puchalski, Christina and Romer, Anna; Taking a Spiritual History allows clinicians to understand patients more fully. Journal of Palliative Medicine Vol 3 No. 1, 2000 p.129

Christina Puchalski; Spiritual Assessment in Clinical Practice; Psychiatric Annals; March 2006; 36,3; Psychology Module pg. 152 (Ehman)

Baranowsky, A. B. (2002). The silencing response in clinical practice. In C. R. Figley (Ed.). *Treating compassion fatigue*. New York: Brunner-Routledge.

Burkhardt, M. A., & Nagai-Jacobson, M. G. (2002). *Spirituality: Living our connectedness*. Albany, NY: Delmar.

Goldberg, B. (1998). Connection: An exploration of spirituality in nursing care. *Journal of Advanced Nursing, 27*, 836-842.

Reed, P. (1992). An emerging paradigm for the investigation of spirituality in nursing. *Research in Nursing & Health, 15*, 349-357.

Taylor, E. J. (2003). Nurses Caring for the Spirit: Patients with Cancer and Family Caregiver Expectations, *Oncology Nursing Forum, 30*, 585-590.

Taylor, E. J. (2002). *Spiritual care: Nursing theory, research, and practice*. Upper Saddle River NJ: Prentice Hall.

Walton, J. (1996). Spiritual relationships. *Journal of Holistic Nursing, 14*, 3.

Breitbart, W., Gibson, C., Poppito, SR, Berg, A. (2004). Psychotherapeutic interventions at the end of life: A focus on meaning and spirituality. *Canadian Journal of Psychiatry, 49*, 366-372.

Byock, I. (1996). The nature of suffering and the nature of opportunity at the end of life. *Clinics in Geriatric Medicine, 12*, 237-252.

Puchalski, C.M. (2002). Spirituality and end of life care: A time for listening and caring. *Journal of Palliative Medicine, 5*, 289-294.

Reed, P. (1992). An Emerging Paradigm for the Investigation of spirituality in nursing. *Research in Nursing and Health*, 15, 349-57

Rumbold, B.D. (2003). Caring for the spirit: Lessons from working with the dying. *Medical Journal of Australia, 179*(6 Suppl), S11-S13.

Festa, L. M., & Tuck, I. (2000). A review of forgiveness literature with implications for nursing practice. *Holistic Nursing Practice, 14,* 77-86.

Halstead, M. & Nilssen, H. (in press). Spiritual care of the older adult with cancer: An evidence-based review of spirituality and health. In D. Cope & A. Reb (Eds.), *An evidence-based approach to the treatment and care of the older adult with cancer.* Pittsburgh, PA:Oncology Nursing Society.

Stoll, R.I. (1989). The essence of spirituality. In V.B. Carson (Ed.). *Spiritual Dimensions of Nursing Practice* (pp. 4-23). Philadelphia: Saunders.

Tanyi, R.A. (2002). Towards clarification of the meaning of spirituality. *Journal of Advanced Nursing,* 39(5), 500-9.

Stoll, R.I. (1983). Emotional and spiritual support. In T.C. Kravis & C.G. Warner (Eds.). *Emergency medicine: A comprehensive review.* Rockville, MD: Aspen.

Mickley, J. & Cowles, K. (2001). Ameliorating the tension: Use of forgiveness for healing. *Oncology Nursing Forum, 28, 31-37.*

Ballard A., Green, T., Logsdon, C. (1997). A comparison of the levels of hope in patients with newly diagnosed and recurrent cancer. *Oncology Nursing Forum, 24(5): 899-904*

Chapman, K. & Pepler, C. (1998). Coping, hope, and anticipatory grief in family members in palliative care. *Cancer Nursing,* 21(4) 226-234.

Ersek, M. (2001). The meaning of hope in the dying,. In B. Ferrell & N. Coyle (Eds.) *Oxford Textbook of Palliative Nursing* (pp. 339-351). New York : Oxford U University Press.

Felder, B. (2004). Hope and coping in patients with cancer diagnoses. *Cancer Nursing ,* 2 27(4), 320-324.

Herth, K. (1990). Fostering hope in terminally-ill people. *Journal of Advanced Nursing,* 15, 1250-1259.

Koopmeiners, L., Post-White, J., Gutjnecht, S., Geransky, C., Nickelson, L., Drew, D., Mackay, K., & Kreitzer, M. (1997). How healthcare professionals contribute to hope in patients with cancer. *Oncology Nursing Forum, 24,* 1507-1513.

Mackey, K., & Kreitzer, M. (1997). How healthcare professionals contribute to h hope in patients with cancer. *Oncology Nursing Forum, 24* (9), 1507-1513.

Miller, J. (1985). Inspiring hope. *American Journal of Nursing. 85, 22-25.*

Poncar, P. (1994). Inspiring hope in the oncology patient. *Journal of Psychosocial N Nursing, 32* (1), 33-38.

Post-White, J., Ceronsky, V., Kreitzer, M., Nickelson, K., Drew, D., Mackey, K., K Koopmeiners, L., & Gutknecht, S. (1996). Hope, spirituality, sense of coherence, and quality of life in patients with cancer. *Oncology Nursing Forum, 23(10),* 1571-1579.

Cassell, E. J. (1991). *The nature of suffering.* New York: Oxford University Press.

Coward, D. C. (1990). The lived experience of self-transcendence in women with advanced breast cancer. *Nursing Science Quarterly, 3,* 162-169.

Eifried, S. (1998). Helping patients find meaning: A caring response to suffering. *International Journal for Human Caring, 2*(1), 33-39.

Eifried, S. (2003). Bearing witness to suffering: The lived experience of nursing students. *Journal of Nursing Education, 42,* 56-67

Eriksson, K. (1997). Caring, spirituality and suffering. In M. S. Roach (Ed.), *Caring from the heart: The convergence of caring and spirituality* (pp. 68-84). New York: Paulist Press.

Ferrell B. R. (1996). *Suffering.* Boston: Jones & Bartlett.

Frank, A. W. (1991). *At the will of the body.* New York: Houghton Mifflin.

Frankl, V. E. (1985). *Man's search for meaning.* New York: Washington Square Press.

Frankl, V. E. (1986). *The doctor and the soul* (3rd Ed.). New York: Vintage

Georges, J. M. (2002). Suffering: Toward a contextual praxis. *Advances in Nursing Science, 25*(1), 79-86.

Gover, I. (2000). Spiritual care in nursing: A systematic approach. *Nursing Standard,* 14, 32-40

Johnson, E. E. (2006). This is about difference. *The Journal of Pastoral Care & Counseling,* 311-314.

Kahn, D. L., & Steeves, R. H. (1986). The experience of suffering: Conceptual clarification and theoretical definition. *Journal of Advanced Nursing,* 11, 623-631.

Kahn, D. L. & Steeves, R. H. (1994). Witnesses to suffering. Nursing knowledge, voice, and vision. *Nursing Outlook,* 42, 260-264.

Kahn, D. L. & Steeves, R. H. (1995). The significance of suffering in cancer care. *Seminars in Oncology Nursing,* 11(1), 9-16.

Lehman, D., Fenza, P., & Hollinger-Smith, L. (2001, May). *Diversity & Cultural Competency in Health Care Settings.* Retrieved from Mather LifeWays: www.matherlifeways.com

Lewis, F. M. (1982). Experienced personal control and quality of life in late-state cancer pages. Nursing Research, 31, 113-119.

Morse, J. M. (2000). Responding to the cues of suffering. *Health Care for Women International,* 21, 1-9.

Morse, J. M. (2001). Toward a praxis theory of suffering. *Advances in Nursing Science, 24*(1), 47-59.

John Patton. (2005). *Pastoral Care: An Essential Guide.* Nashville: Abingdon Press

Picard, C. (1991). Caring and the story: The compelling nature of what must be told and understood in the human dimension of suffering. In D. A. Gaut & M. M. Leininger (Eds.), *Caring: The compassionate healer* (pp. 89-98). New York: National League for Nursing Press.

Rawlinson, M. C. (1986). The sense of suffering. *The Journal of Medicine and Philosophy*, 11, 39-62.

Jewish Outreach Institute. (2008). Retrieved October 15, 2012, from Jewish Outreach Institute: http://www.joi.org/qa/denom.shtml

Remen, R. N. (2006). *Kitchen Table Wisdom: Stories that Heal*. New York: The Penguin Group.

Rosen, R. (2000). *Global Literacies: Lesson on Business Leadership and National Cultures*. New York: Simon & Schuster.

Spencer-Oatey, H. (2000). *Culturally Speaking: Mananging Rapport through Talk across Cultures*. London: Continuum.

Rodgers, B. L., & Cowles, K. V. (1997). A conceptual foundation for human suffering in nursing care and research. *Journal of Advanced Nursing*, 25, 1048-1053

Rowe, J. (2003). The suffering of the healer. *Nursing Forum, 38*(4), 16-20.

Starck, P. L., & McGovern, J. P. (1992). *The hidden dimension of illness: Human suffering*. New York: National League for Nursing Press.

Taylor, Elizabeth J. (2002). *Spiritual Care: Nursing Theory, Research, and Practice*. New Jersey: Pearson Education, Inc.

Amenta, M.O. (1986). Spiritual Concerns (Chapter 9, pp. 115 – 161). In M.O. Amenta & N. Bohnet (Eds.). *Nursing care of the terminally ill*. Boston: Little, Brown.

Steeves, R. H. (1992). Patients who have undergone bone marrow transplantation: Their quest for meaning. *Oncology Nursing Forum*, 19, 899-905.

Fowler, M., & Peterson, B.S. (1997). Spiritual themes in clinical pastoral education. *Journal of Training and Supervision in Ministry*, 18, 46-54

Steeves, R., Cohen, M. Z., & Wise, C. T. (1994). An analysis of critical incidents describing the essence of oncology nursing. *Oncology Nursing Forum, 21*(8, Supplement), 19-25.

Dombeck, M.B. (1996). Chaos and self-organization as a consequence of spiritual disequilibrium. *Clinical Nurse Specialist*. 10(2), 69-75.

Steeves, R. H., & Kahn, D. L. (1987). Experience of meaning in suffering. *Image*, 19, 114-116.

Dossey, B.M., & Guzzetta, C.E. (2000). Holistic nursing practice. In B.M. Dossey, L. Keegan, & C.E. Guzzetta (Eds.), *Holistic nursing: A handbook for practice* (3rd ed., pp. 5-26), Rockville, MD: Aspen.

Susan Wintz, Earl Cooper. (2009). *Cultural & Spiritual Sensitivity: A learning module for health care professionals.*

Tapp, D. M. (2001). Conserving the vitality of suffering: Addressing family constraints to illness conversations. *Nursing inquiry*, 8(4), 254-263.

Taylor, E. J. (1993). Factors associated with meaning in life among people with recurrent cancer. *Oncology Nursing Forum*, 20, 1399-1407.

Ferrell, B.R., Grant, M., Funk, B., Garcia, N., Otis-Green, S., & Schaffner, M.L.J. (1996). Quality of life in breast cancer. *Cancer practice*, 4, 331-340.

Kolatch, Alfred J. *The Jewish Book of Why/The Second Jewish Book of Why*. NY: Jonathan David Publishers, 1989.

Mauk, Kristen L., Schmidt, Nola K. (2004). *Spiritual Care in Nursing Practice.* Philadelphia: Lippincott Williams & Wilkins.

O'Brien, M.E. (1999). *Spirituality in nursing: Standing on holy ground*. Sudbury, MA: Jones and Bartlett.

McSherry, Wilfred. (2007). The Meaning of Spirituality and Spiritual Care within Nursing and Health care Practice. London: MA Healthcare Ltd

Jewish Outreach Institute. (2008). Retrieved October 15, 2012, from Jewish Outreach Institute: http://www.joi.org/qa/denom.shtml

The George H Gallup International Institute. Spiritual beliefs and the dying process, a report of a national survey conducted for the Nathan Cummings Foundation and Fetzer Institute.

Princeton, NJ: The George H Gallup International Institute; October 1997:1.

Wells, M. (2000). Beyond cultural competence: A model for individual and institutional cultural development. *Journal for Community Health Nurses*, 189-99.

CPSIA information can be obtained
at www.ICGtesting.com
Printed in the USA
LVOW03s2325280118
564397LV00001B/60/P

9 781682 566824